LOSE IT
FOREVER

Also by Jason Karp

The Inner Runner

Run Your Fat Off

Sexercise

Running for Women

Running a Marathon For Dummies

14-Minute Metabolic Workouts

101 Winning Racing Strategies for Runners

*101 Developmental Concepts &
Workouts for Cross Country Runners*

How to Survive Your PhD

LOSE IT
FOREVER

**The 6 Habits of Successful Weight Losers
from the National Weight Control Registry**

JASON R. KARP, PHD

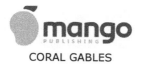

CORAL GABLES

Cover Design: Jayoung Hong
Cover Photo: Adobe Stock/ Tatiana Plotnikova
Layout Design: Jayoung Hong

Notice: The author and publisher specifically disclaim all responsibility for any injury, liability, loss, or risk, personal or otherwise, that is incurred as a consequence, directly or indirectly, of the use and application of any of the contents of this book. Before starting any exercise program, please obtain the approval from a qualified medical professional.

For permission requests, please contact the publisher at:
Mango Publishing Group
2850 S Douglas Road, 2nd Floor
Coral Gables, FL 33134 USA
info@mango.bz

For special orders, quantity sales, course adoptions and corporate sales, please email the publisher at sales@mango.bz. For trade and wholesale sales, please contact Ingram Publisher Services at customer.service@ingramcontent.com or +1.800.509.4887.

Lose It Forever: The 6 Habits of Successful Weight Losers from the National Weight Control Registry

Library of Congress Cataloging-in-Publication number has been requested
ISBN: (p) 978-1-64250-346-3 (e) 978-1-64250-347-0
BISAC category code HEA010000, HEALTH & FITNESS / Healthy Living

Printed in the United States of America

To my parents,
Muriel and Monroe,
for the habits they instilled in me

Table of Contents

WARM-UP

In a national television interview with Barbara Walters in 2014, Oprah Winfrey confessed that not being able to maintain her weight loss was her biggest regret. In that interview, Walters asked Winfrey to finish the sentence, "Before I leave this Earth, I will not be satisfied until I..."

"Until I make peace with the whole weight thing," Oprah replied.

Losing weight is hard; keeping it off is even harder. Dr. Albert Stunkard and Mavis McLaren-Hume of the Departments of Psychiatry and Medicine of the University of Pennsylvania School of Medicine and the Nutrition Clinic of the New York Hospital may have been the first researchers to study just how hard it is. For their research, which was published in 1959 in the prestigious journal, *Archives of Internal Medicine*, they followed one hundred obese individuals in the Nutrition Clinic of the New York Hospital. Two years after treatment, they discovered that only 2 percent maintained a weight loss of at least twenty pounds.[1] This finding was instrumental in creating the perception, which has been perpetuated in popular media and by celebrities' well-documented yo-yo dieting and weight fluctuations, that hardly anyone succeeds in keeping the weight off.

The field of medicine is often stuck on studying failures, focusing on people who fail and then concluding that the failures represent reality. Although success rates are low, keeping weight off is not as rare as Stunkard and Mavis' report or Oprah Winfrey's regrets have led people to believe. The difficulty in maintaining weight loss is due (mostly) to behavioral factors—specifically, the difficulty in making permanent changes in your lifestyle.

How hard is it to change your behaviors? As Oprah and millions of other unsuccessful weight losers have shown, it's pretty hard. Three-quarters of Americans say they have tried to lose weight at some point in their lives, and 20 percent of people who are obese have tried at least twenty times to lose weight.[2] Most people in behavioral weight-loss programs lose about 10 percent of their weight over twenty to twenty-four weeks, but, within just one year, they regain an average of one-third of their weight loss and return to their pre-weight-loss weight within three to five years.[3,4] It takes specific behaviors to prevent this weight regain from happening. Those behaviors become habits if they are repeatedly practiced over time within highly similar contexts.[5]

Most of us have habits. Some of our habits may lead us to be effective and successful, and some of our habits may lead us to be ineffective and unsuccessful. Some of us may roll the toilet paper from the top and some from the bottom. Other habits—both positive and negative—have much greater consequences. Changing those habits, or at least modifying them to achieve your goals, can be difficult, especially with age. The older you get, the more "you" you become. And so habits that led you to become overweight also lead you to remain overweight, especially as you age. As physicist Isaac Newton taught, a body in motion stays in motion, unless acted on by an unequal force. To change your motion, you need an unequal force.

Habits don't become habits overnight. When we get excited about doing something, it's easy to jump in and, in the words of Nike, just do it. But that strategy often fails in the long term because "just doing it" doesn't always, or even usually, make a behavior stick. That takes persistence. To be persistent, you need to create the environment for the behaviors to become automatic and become habits. It often takes months or even years to make permanent changes. Many successful weight losers fail many times at keeping their weight off before finally succeeding. All those failed attempts are not really failures, because they created the opportunity for the successful attempt. It takes many tries at doing something over and over and over again before the actions become habitual. Think about the last time you drove your car. Did you have to consciously think about where to put your hands on the steering wheel? What about when to press on the brake or look in the rearview mirror? But you had to bring a certain consciousness to all those things when you first learned to drive a car as a teenager. Driving a car wasn't a habit back then. It took many attempts at driving a car for it to become a habit. Driving becomes such a habit that, oftentimes, we don't even know how we got to our destination!

Seventy-five percent of Americans (and 81 percent of obese Americans) perceive lack of willpower as the biggest barrier to successful weight loss.[6] But, according to psychologist Wendy Wood, PhD, it's a myth that behavior change is all about a strong intention and the willpower to implement it. Rather, her research suggests, behavior change is about forming habits.[7] Habits go beyond intention and willpower; they are automatic behaviors. Most people don't consciously set the intention to brush their teeth every day; they just do. Becoming a successful weight loser requires exactly the same approach: creating the habits to keep your weight off, so that your actions become automatic. Dr. Wood says that when we repeat an action over and over again in a given context and then get a reward for doing so, we are learning very slowly and incrementally to associate that context with that behavior.

In other words, habits have a life of their own, because, once formed, they stop being conscious and become automatic.

Once you have formed a desirable habit, however, that doesn't mean it can't be undone. It can be undone, because the undesirable habit is never unlearned; it is just replaced by a new, desirable habit. In the face of the stimulus that caused the undesirable habit, it's relatively easy for that undesirable habit to reemerge; old habits really do die hard. Therefore, desirable habits need to be constantly reinforced, while undesirable habits need to be constantly suppressed. Your chances of becoming a successful weight loser will be considerably improved by focusing on both the reinforcement of desirable habits and on the suppression of undesirable habits.

And that's how most diets fail. After months of sticking to a specific way of eating, all it takes is one reintroduction of a previously conditioned stimulus to fall off the wagon and revert to the undesirable habit. Most diets and weight-loss plans are short-term fixes to a long-term problem. They lure you with promises of quick, dramatic results, like "lose ten pounds in ten days." They don't emphasize the critical aspect of being able to *maintain* weight beyond those ten days and for the next ten years or more. But everyone who loses weight wants to keep it off. After all, there's little point to losing weight if you're just going to regain it. Popular diets don't teach you the habits or provide you with strategies to keep the weight off. Perhaps they don't do that because that's not the sexy, alluring part of weight loss. It's alluring to say that you can lose ten pounds in ten days. And it's even possible that you can. Weight loss, especially rapid weight loss, is exciting. There's not much that's exciting about maintaining weight, even though it's more important. But, you'll almost surely gain back those ten pounds, unless you have developed the habits and have a system in place to prevent that from happening.

Being overweight negatively impacts your physical and mental health. It impacts how you live your life. It creates a lot of unhappiness. Research has shown that negative attitudes about body weight—called internalized weight bias—cause a devalued sense of self-worth.[8] Perhaps not surprisingly, women typically have greater internalized weight bias than men. Body mass index, the most common measure of obesity, is positively correlated with weight bias—the greater the weight bias, the higher the body mass index. Having less weight bias is associated with maintenance of greater weight loss, and weight bias predicts who will regain weight. Successful weight losers have less internalized weight bias compared to people who gain their weight back.

If being overweight is bad for your physical and mental health, it's not surprising that losing weight has the opposite consequences. Losing just 5 to 10 percent of your body weight confers a wide range of health benefits, from a substantially reduced risk for cardiovascular disease and diabetes and lower blood pressure and cholesterol to less depression and anxiety and better cognitive function. Losing weight also decreases the risk of certain types of cancer, enhances sleep, gives you a better sex life, ameliorates symptoms of depression, and even, perhaps, helps you live longer.

While it may seem obvious, perhaps the greatest benefit of losing weight and keeping it off is that you'll look better. That may sound superficial, but looking better makes you feel good about yourself. And feeling good about yourself has wide-reaching ramifications, including strengthening your belief in yourself and in what you can accomplish. Losing weight can fill the hole created by insecurity. Why it does so, at least in my view, is because humans, like all animals, are physical beings. We live through our bodies. Because we live a physical life, our identity and self-worth are often intimately connected to our physical presence. Most of us have witnessed the athlete who walks with a swagger, bespeaking the confidence that lies beneath. Self-worth is arguably the most important factor in determining what actions and directions people take in their lives. To extend René Descartes' maxim, I think, therefore I am what I think I am.

Contrary to other weight-loss books, *Lose It Forever* shares the habits of the people who have maintained their weight loss over the long term, from the research that has scientifically measured it. This distinction between weight loss and weight maintenance is critical, because what you need to do to keep the weight off in the long term is different from what you need to do to lose weight in the first place. To lose it forever, you need to create habits. You can do it if you persevere.

INTRODUCTION

"I INTUITIVELY KNEW THAT ANYTHING I DID WOULD HAVE TO BECOME PART OF MY LIFESTYLE INDEFINITELY."

On Monday morning, forty-eight-year-old Lynn Kata stands on one leg and squats on a *Wii Fit* Balance Board in her living room. The exercise video game, a gift she requested for Mother's Day, includes more than forty exercise activities, including yoga, strength training, aerobics, and balance games. As she follows the fitness trainer demonstrating the exercises on the screen, the balance board detects and tracks Lynn's center of balance and measures her weight. At 155 pounds, she is told by the game's avatar that she is overweight.

An active child and teenager in the Chicago suburb of Oak Lawn, Lynn was on the Pom Pom Squad in high school and spent her summers taking gymnastics classes. After high school, she spent a good part of her late teens and early twenties working, attending college classes, and going out with her friends to dance in local discos. She took dance lessons and joined the local dance troupe *Dance Mania* when she was twenty years old. "Dancing had always been an enjoyable part of my life and kept me in really good shape," she says. As a young adult, life was good. She graduated from college in 1986 with a degree in media management, got married in 1987, moved to Crestwood, Illinois, and had her first child in 1988. A second child came two years later. She lost her baby weight and became a busy stay-at-home mom.

In 1991, Lynn quit smoking and gained ten pounds. After Lynn's third child was born when she was thirty-seven, she was unable to get back to her pre-baby weight. "I wasn't a dieter, so I just settled in with the extra weight," she says. For years, she kept busy as a mom, serving as the choreographer for her kids' school's annual fashion show fundraiser and teaching art classes at their school. "I loved being a mom and was very active in my kids' school and sports activities," she says. She continued to eat what she had always eaten—meat, dairy, and processed carbs. During the next several years, she gained another twenty pounds.

In May 2008, at age forty-eight, she decided to leave teaching and pursue other opportunities. "The photos from my going-away party were my wake-up call," she says. "I was shocked by my appearance. I knew I had gained weight because I had to keep buying bigger clothes, but, in my mind, I was still a normal-weight person. Those photos showed me someone I didn't recognize as myself. I decided it was time for a change." Lynn made herself a promise that she was going to lose the extra weight for her fiftieth birthday, which was a year and a half away.

***

Your coworker's sister's husband can make you fat, even if you don't know him. Such was the discovery of Yale physician and sociologist Nicholas Christakis, MD, PhD, whose fascinating work at Harvard University revealed that obesity, much like the spread of a disease, can spread through social networks. Dr. Christakis found that the risk of obesity among acquaintances or friends of an obese individual was 45 percent higher in a connected network of people than in a random network.[9] Specifically, the risk of obesity was about 20 percent higher for an obese individual's friend's friends (two degrees of separation) and about 10 percent higher for the obese individual's friends' friends' friends (three degrees of separation). By the fourth degree of separation, like your coworker's sister's husband's bowling partner, there was no longer a relationship between an individual's obesity and the fourth-degree person's obesity. Dr. Christakis also found that relational distance plays a stronger role in the spread of obesity than even geographic distance, so it doesn't seem to matter if your colleague's sister's husband lives anywhere near you. Studying obesity within families, Dr. Christakis found among pairs of adult siblings that one sibling's chance of becoming obese increased by 40 percent if the other sibling became obese. This phenomenon was more marked among siblings of the same sex than among siblings of the opposite sex. Same-sex mutual friends also have the strongest influence on each other's weight gain. Among married couples, when either the husband or wife becomes obese, the other spouse is 37 percent more likely to become obese. The opposite phenomenon also seems to be true: to lose weight, weight-loss interventions that modify the overweight person's social network are more successful than those that don't. In other words, if you want to lose weight, it's beneficial to hang around thin people.

But just picking the right friends and relatives isn't enough to *stay* slim. Since most people who go on a diet and lose weight gain the weight back, the only reliable proof of what works for permanent weight loss comes from the people who have actually achieved permanent weight loss. What is unique about those who succeed? And how can you succeed like them?

The answer is buried deep in the archives at the Weight Control and Diabetes Research Center in Providence, Rhode Island: the National Weight Control Registry (NWCR), the largest database ever assembled on individuals successful at long-term maintenance of weight loss. Founded in 1994 by Rena Wing,

PhD, Professor of Psychiatry and Human Behavior at Brown Medical School and director of the Weight Control & Diabetes Research Center at The Miriam Hospital, and James Hill, PhD, chair of the Department of Nutrition Sciences and director of the Nutrition Obesity Research Center at the University of Alabama, Birmingham (formerly professor of Pediatrics and Medicine at the University of Colorado Health Sciences Center at the time he cofounded the NWCR), the NWCR includes more than 10,000 individuals who complete annual questionnaires about their current weight, diet, exercise habits, and behavioral strategies for weight-loss maintenance. The goal of the NWCR, which started with ninety-two people enrolled in its first year,[10] is to identify the behaviors used by successful weight losers to help others become successful weight losers. According to Drs. Wing and Hill, part of the reason for developing the registry was to counter the belief that no one succeeds long-term at weight loss.[11]

The NWCR is a gold mine of successful weight-loss information, containing extensive data on individuals who have lost at least thirty pounds (which represents a minimum 10 percent weight loss for most overweight and obese individuals) and have maintained a weight loss of at least thirty pounds for at least one year.

Who are the people in the NWCR? Eighty percent are women and 20 percent are men. The average woman is forty-five years old and weighs 145 pounds, while the average man is forty-nine years old and weighs 190 pounds. Ninety-five percent of members are Caucasian, 64 percent are married, and 61 percent have a bachelor's degree or higher. Forty-five percent lost the weight on their own and 55 percent lost the weight with the help of a formal weight-loss program. Before becoming successful weight losers, 90 percent of NWCR members had failed at keeping their weight off, many failing multiple times. They had also struggled with their weight for a long time—46 percent became overweight before the age of twelve, and 72 percent became overweight before the age of eighteen. Forty-six percent have one parent who is overweight or obese, and 27 percent have both parents overweight or obese.

The average weight loss of the NWCR members upon entry into the registry is 68.9 pounds (which decreased their body mass index from 35 to 25 kg/m^2), kept off for an average of five and a half years. Although these average numbers are impressive, they hide a lot of diversity: NWCR weight losses range from thirty to three hundred pounds, nearly 20 percent have lost at least one hundred pounds, and the duration of successful weight loss ranges from one year to sixty-six years!

To date, thirty-nine scientific papers have been published using the data from the NWCR on the strategies and habits of successful weight losers, characteristics associated with weight-loss maintenance, and the risk factors of weight regain. The earliest of these studies, which was published in *American Journal of Clinical Nutrition* in 1997, described some of the basic habits of 629 female and 155 male members.[12] The researchers found that 55 percent (60 percent of women and 37 percent of men) used a formal weight-loss program or professional assistance to lose weight, and 89 percent modified both their diet and physical activity to lose weight.

From this initial descriptive study has grown dozens of studies that have delved into the habits of the largest database of successful weight losers. When individuals enroll in the NWCR, they're asked to complete several questionnaires that detail how they initially lost weight and how they maintain their weight loss. They are tracked yearly to determine changes in their weight and in their weight-related behaviors.

In one of the earlier NWCR studies, which included 893 members (81 percent women, 19 percent men; average age of forty-four), 447 said they lost weight on their own, 313 said they lost weight through an organized program (e.g., Weight Watchers, Jenny Craig, etc.), and 133 said they lost weight through a formal program that used a liquid formula diet (e.g., Optifast, New Directions, etc.).[13] Those who used a liquid formula diet to lose weight relied more heavily than the others on specific dietary strategies, such as counting calories, limiting percentage of calories from fat, and limiting the quantities of foods consumed. Individuals who lost weight on their own were more likely to be male and have less history of weight cycling. These individuals were more likely to weigh themselves at least once a week, suggesting that weighing may be an important part of their self-regulation of body weight. Those who lost weight on their own expended a greater number of calories through strenuous activities than the others. These individuals were more likely to regulate their body weight through exercise rather than diet. A later study on 2,964 NWCR members compared young adults (eighteen to thirty-five years old) and older adults (thirty-six to fifty years old) to see if there are age-based differences in approaches to weight loss.[14] Young adults placed greater emphasis on physical appearance and social factors for losing weight and less emphasis on their health compared to older adults. They also were more likely than older adults to take exercise classes and to lose weight on their own without help and were less likely to use a commercial weight-loss program.

Because it's so common for weight losers to gain the weight back, many of the NWCR studies have examined the factors that contribute to and even predict weight regain.[15-20] Believe it or not, whether or not you regain weight after losing it is predictable. Not surprisingly, a greater amount of initial weight loss is a predictor of weight regain. It's harder to keep off eighty pounds than to keep off thirty pounds. One of the NWCR studies found that individuals who had lost 30 percent or more of their maximum lifetime weight at the time they entered the registry had a greater risk of gaining weight after one year compared to those who lost less than 25 percent of their maximum weight.[21] Several other factors that predict which individuals would gain weight versus those who would remain successful weight losers include weighing more to begin with, a shorter duration of weight-loss maintenance, a greater history of weight cycling (many ups and downs of weight), dietary disinhibition, binge eating, depression, and several eating and exercise behaviors (e.g., increased caloric intake, TV watching, and decreased physical activity). If consuming many daily calories, watching TV, and not exercising are habits that are toxic, leading to weight regain and unsuccessful weight loss, the opposite habits are tonic, leading to successful, permanent weight loss.

Although very successful, the members of the NWCR are not superheroes who are immune to the pitfalls that cause weight regain. Like other weight losers, many NWCR members have regained weight. One year after entering the registry, 35 percent gained five pounds or more, with an average weight gain of 15.5 pounds. However, 59 percent have maintained their weight loss, and 6 percent have lost additional weight. Weight trajectories are curvilinear, with more rapid regain early and very little regain after five years. Heavier individuals have regained weight more quickly initially, but have maintained significantly greater weight losses over ten years. Encouragingly, 88 percent have maintained a weight loss of at least 10 percent of their lifetime maximum body weight for five years and 87 percent for ten years, with weight losses averaging 52.4 pounds (23.8 kg) after five years and 50.8 pounds (23.1 kg) after ten years.[22]

It often takes a catastrophic event or trigger to change behavior. A medical trigger is one such event, because it threatens our health. People who have medical triggers for losing weight lose more weight and are more successful at maintaining their weight loss than those with nonmedical triggers for losing weight or no trigger at all. That was the conclusion of a NWCR study, published in the journal *Preventive Medicine* in 2004, that asked 917 NWCR members (average age of 46.6 years) if there were a specific incident or triggering event that prompted them to begin their successful weight loss and, if yes, to select from multiple options what type of event it was (medical, emotional, lifestyle, inspiration or impetus from another person, weight-loss program became available, saw picture or image of self, reached lifetime high weight or size).[23] Changes in body weight over two years were compared between three groups: (1) those who had medical triggers, (2) those who had nonmedical triggers, and (3) those who had no trigger for weight loss. Eighty-three percent of NWCR members had a trigger to lose weight, with a medical trigger being the most common (23 percent). Those with a medical trigger lost significantly more weight (80.3 pounds) compared to those with nonmedical triggers (70 pounds) or no triggers (70 pounds). In addition, members with a medical trigger regained significantly less weight after one and two years compared to those with nonmedical triggers and no trigger. A medical trigger can be a powerful initiator of behavior change.

As much of a gold mine of information that the NWCR is, it's not without its limitations or criticisms. For starters, its members are not randomly selected from the general population. They are self-selected, volunteering to become members of the NWCR after seeing an advertisement for it or discovering it on their own. As a result, the registry's members are not a representative sample of the population of weight losers or dieters. It's possible that individuals who are the most successful at weight loss may be more inclined to join the NWCR. Therefore, the results of the NWCR research have limited generalizability to the entire population of overweight and obese individuals. The NWCR should not be viewed as a magic formula for successful weight loss for everyone.

Another limitation is that nearly all the data on the NWCR members have been collected via questionnaires that are sent to them, in the early years via mail and, in more recent years, via email. In questionnaire-based research, individuals report on the studied variables themselves, rather than those variables being directly measured by the researchers (for example, if I ask you to tell me how much you weigh instead of weighing you myself). This necessitates a good memory and the ability to estimate things, like the amount of food eaten and the amount and intensity of exercise done. While some self-reported variables are generally accurate, like body weight and height, other variables, like caloric intake and amount of exercise, are subject to larger errors. Most people underestimate how many calories they consume and overestimate how much they exercise. Questionnaires are also subject to a response bias. For example, individuals more likely to regain weight after joining the NWCR may choose not to answer the follow-up questionnaires, perhaps because they are embarrassed or otherwise don't want to admit their failures. It would be virtually impossible to directly measure every studied variable on each member of the NWCR, especially when many of the variables are retrospective in nature (e.g., an individual's maximum lifetime weight, number of years having kept the weight off, or how many minutes of exercise done last week).

The large sample sizes of the NWCR studies, which are in the hundreds and even thousands, help to alleviate (but not eliminate) these limitations, and are major strengths of the studies, since sample size is one of the main factors that affects the statistical power of scientific research. To try to get around the self-selection limitation, the founders of the NWCR also did some research outside of their database. To determine whether there are characteristics of successful weight losers in a population-based sample (compared to the self-selected sample of the NWCR) that distinguish them from unsuccessful weight losers and from never-overweight individuals, the scientists of the NWCR made some phone calls—2,382 to be exact—to people in the community, which resulted in 500 completed calls and data from 238 people to be analyzed.[24] These 238 people were divided into three groups: (1) successful weight losers (those who had intentionally lost at least 10 percent of their maximum weight at some point in their lives, were currently at least 10 percent below their maximum weight, and had maintained at least 10 percent weight loss for at least one year); (2) weight-loss regainers (those who had intentionally lost at least 10 percent of their maximum weight, but were not currently at least 10 percent below their maximum weight), and (3) weight-stable individuals (those who had never lost 10 percent of their maximum weight, were never at least 10 percent above their current weight, and had maintained their current weight within ten pounds for the past five years). The scientists discovered that 21 percent of this random, population-based sample were successful weight losers and, even more interesting, they had similar habits to keep the weight off as did the members of the NWCR. The study's results contrast sharply with the popular belief that no one ever succeeds in losing weight or maintaining their weight loss. This finding, and others like it, hold out the promise that weight regain is not inevitable, and that people can recover from even the most severe weight gain. The good news, then, is that behaviors as profound as those causing obesity can change, and that the route to such change is through the creation of habits.

The research from the NWCR has been largely ignored by those who can make a difference—medical professionals, fitness professionals, weight-loss coaches, even social media influencers and your next-door neighbor. When was the last time you saw research from the NWCR posted on Instagram or Facebook? Unfortunately, the general public does not read scientific journals and so is not aware of the information. Shockingly, no one has written a book to introduce the data and give practical advice based on it. That's horrible, because the public needs to know! *Lose It Forever* does just that. In the pages that follow, you'll find the pertinent data and learn what other people in the same position have done, and continue to do, to keep their weight off.

Given the plethora of weight-loss programs, books, social media anecdotes, and next-door neighbor accounts, it's clear that there are many ways to lose weight. You may know someone who lost weight by eating less fat or less carbohydrate, going to the gym, or by adopting a ketogenic diet. Perhaps you have tried one or more ways yourself. An interesting finding of the NWCR research is that, while approaches to *lose weight* differ greatly, with no commonalities in type of diet modification, there is much more similarity in the strategies used to *maintain* weight loss. Successful weight losers act like other successful weight losers. Weight loss and weight maintenance are not the same; they require different strategies. When you review all the data and research on successful weight losers from the NWCR, as well as that from outside of the NWCR, one thing becomes very clear: to be a successful weight loser for the rest of your life, you need to adopt specific behavioral strategies. That's what this book is all about.

Unfortunately, there is no cure for obesity or being overweight. While maintaining lost weight gets easier over time, people still have to work hard to keep the weight off, even fifteen to twenty years after losing it. Behavior is not an easy thing to change. Most of us know how easy it is to get stuck in a rut, doing the same thing over and over again. It's difficult and uncomfortable to do something we're not used to doing. To be a permanent, successful weight loser, it is essential to totally restructure your food and exercise behaviors. Sounds hard, but so is anything in life that is worth doing. In the pages that follow, the successful weight losers of the NWCR show you how.

***

"Since I never followed a diet before, I really had no idea where to start," Lynn Kata says. "Since exercise had kept me in shape before, I was willing to try to get back into moving and burning off some calories." In addition to exercising with *Wii Fit*, she walked about a mile with her dog every morning. "My dog won't leave me alone until I take her for a walk," she says. "It felt good to be outside in the fresh air. It helped my mental health as much as my physical health." She also stopped putting sugar in her coffee and stopped drinking sweetened beverages, including soft drinks and juices, replacing them with carbonated water. It worked. "The first ten pounds came off easily," she says.

Since success often breeds the motivation to do more, Lynn started walking farther. She began walking about three miles around her neighborhood. As she became fitter, she walked faster, adding music for inspiration. "Every morning the *Wii Fit* graph displayed a chart, showing my weight decreasing," she says. "Looking back, I believe the tracking of my progress helped to keep me motivated."

Although Lynn was walking a lot, her diet remained the same. Then she learned that walking one mile burns approximately a hundred calories. "That was an 'aha' moment for me," she says, "because I realized I could wipe out my calorie burn from my one mile walk by eating just one cookie!" As Lynn found out, it's too easy to replace calories after completing a workout—the twenty minutes of walking to burn a hundred calories can indeed be negated in just a few seconds with a cookie, even a healthy one.

Lynn started paying much closer attention to how much she ate, not simply what she ate. "I stopped eating desserts. I cut down on snacks," she says. She lost the weight slowly—about a pound a week, sometimes two weeks, but it worked. Her next goal was to increase the amount of exercise. "I purchased a set of DVDs called *The Lotte Berk Method*, primarily because the picture on the front of the package showed an extremely fit woman," she says. So, Lynn worked out thirty minutes every morning to "Hip Hugger Abs" and "High Round Assets." Her body started transforming back to her younger, fit body. "I loved seeing the progress," she says. Other people began to notice. She bought new clothes to fit her new body and immediately got rid of the clothes that were too big. "There was no going back," she says. "I liked the new me!"

She was offered a job as a front desk attendant at a local health and recreation center. Inspired by that environment, she decided to become a certified group fitness instructor. She heard about a workout called Zumba, a group fitness class that combines dance, music, and a fun atmosphere. She attended a class and was hooked. After getting certified to teach Zumba, she started teaching classes in January 2010. "My first class was attended by over seventy people!" she says. "My fitness career had begun."

When asked about her weight loss, Lynn says, "I didn't know specifically what I should do, so I just came up with my own method. It was a learning process to figure out what would work for me. I wasn't interested in trying out any fad diets or pre-packaged meals. I wasn't interested in using supplements or pills. I intuitively knew that anything I did would have to become part of my lifestyle indefinitely. I knew too many people who had tried those other methods and were unable to sustain their weight loss. I believe now that sustainable changes that slowly became my new normal were the key to my success."

Ten years later, Lynn still walks every day and teaches Zumba classes at the recreation center. She takes Zumba instructor courses to learn new formats and attends Zumba conventions. She has even taught Zumba on Celebrity Cruise lines, traveling to Europe and the Caribbean, and was cast as a Zumba class participant on an episode of the TV show, *Chicago Fire* in 2014.

Now sixty years old, Lynn weighs 115 pounds. She has lost a total of forty pounds and has maintained that forty-pound weight loss for more than ten years, avoiding the yo-yo dieting that is so common among weight losers. She joined the NWCR in 2012 because she was interested to find out how the registry helps people gain the knowledge they need to maintain their weight loss. After submitting her success story to the NWCR, she was contacted by a few national publications and news outlets, and even had an article published about her weight loss in *Better Homes and Gardens*. She became a National Board-Certified Health Coach in 2017 to help others set achievable goals and hold them accountable. "I now know that being healthy is not just about moving your body and eating healthy food, but also about creating a lifestyle and habits that support health and happiness," she says. "'Eat less, move more' is a catchy phrase, but some people need help creating those habits."

Lynn's successful weight maintenance habits include weighing herself every day, educating herself on healthy eating, eating more fruit, vegetables, whole grains, nuts, seeds, and legumes, and eating less meat, dairy, processed carbs, unhealthy fats, and sugar. She still walks every day, which is the most common exercise of the NWCR. She doesn't drink sweetened beverages and doesn't eat sweets.

Working at a fitness facility, Lynn sees many people whose workouts are so ambitious and unsustainable that they quit. "Most people go all-out for a few days or weeks in January and then never come back," she says. When asked what advice she has for others, she says, "Find the physical activities that you enjoy and do them. You have to start small and build. Join a class if you like being in a group environment. You meet people and motivate each other. Or get a workout buddy.

"It's not about the fancy fitness equipment, as anyone who has ever bought a treadmill or other home gym and then used it as a clothes hanger can attest. It's not about the gym memberships that go unused every year. It's not about the latest bestselling book on the newest diet. It's not about dietary supplements that are a short-term solution. It's not about cosmetic medical procedures for a temporary fix. You can buy every gadget or workout DVD being hawked on television that promises quick results and shows amazing before-and-after photos and testimonials. When the disclaimer says, 'Results are not typical,' they're not kidding. Stop kidding yourself. It's about being healthy from the inside out. You have to focus on what your body really needs."

HABIT 1

Live with Intention

"I BURIED MY MOTHER AND MADE AN APPOINTMENT FOR MY FIRST EVER DOCTOR'S VISIT ON THE WAY HOME FROM THE CEMETERY."

In Louisville, Kentucky, forty-five-year-old business organizations and municipal law attorney Jeremy Kirkham stands at his office desk while he talks on the phone with a client. He stands whenever he can. When his phone calls include only listening rather than talking, he briskly walks. As chair of Louisville Metro's Code Enforcement Board, he acts as a Hearing Officer for any noncriminal violations of local ordinances that are appealed by citizens. Although his docket demands that he sit for hours at a time to hear cases, he stands whenever possible.

Unlike the offices of other high-profile professionals, Jeremy's office doesn't overlook any of Louisville's landmarks, like Churchill Downs, the Ohio River, or PNC Tower. In fact, there's not much outside his office window at all, save for some grass, a few leafless trees, and walking paths that wind through the development, and that is very much by design. Jeremy bought an office condo in a park-like development where cars cannot be parked right up against the building. "I purposefully wanted a boiler-room setup that encouraged me to get up and walk out of my office and into the community as much as possible," he says. "When I'm working, I like to keep moving."

Jeremy has been losing weight for a long time. When he was seven years old, his mother put him on his first diet. "From an early age, it was evident that my mother's regard for me was conditioned on my weight," he says. "Initially, I interpreted it the same way I would have any correction from my mother. 'You are fat; you need to lose weight' was on the same level as

'Your shoes are untied; tie your shoes' or 'Your hair is messy; comb your hair.' In all such instances, the identified deficiency was accompanied by Mother's oversight and assistance."

Over time, Jeremy noticed what was different about those other deficiencies. He could tie his shoes and the problem was solved. He could comb his hair and the problem was solved. "Losing weight was different because I never seemed to be able to do it and make it stick," he says. "Eating half a grapefruit before every meal and doing the Jane Fonda workout tape every day didn't work as planned, so constantly having cottage cheese and fruit and doing Richard Simmons workouts became the thing to do." When those methods didn't work, Jeremy was put on a calorie-restriction-during-the-week-and-splurge-on-the-weekends diet. Throughout Jeremy's childhood, his mother put him on a number of different diets and exercise programs, often ones she found in magazines and on television.

With no results that would make his mother happy, his despair increased, along with his resistance. "She raised me alone, and my grandparents shared a significant portion of the burden of raising me," he says. His mother would send him to his grandparents' house with instructions about what he could and could not eat and gave him a list of exercises he was required to do. When she suspected he was not performing the tasks as assigned, she required him to carry a pedometer so she would know he was at least jogging and walking. "One day, after my grandfather took me for a walk in the woods, he treated me to a bowl of butter pecan ice cream. It was customary for Mother to inquire about what I ate when with my grandparents and, when she came to pick me up, I told her the truth. She angrily confronted my grandparents on the spot and threatened to put a stop to my visits if they failed to conform to her wishes concerning my diet."

These experiences influenced the way Jeremy thought about eating. "After several diet and exercise evolutions, I felt that hunger was my enemy because that led to me wanting to eat," he says. "And as a natural consequence of that belief and of the mental conditioning to which I had been exposed, I felt that I was a failure and a disappointment as a person and as a son because I couldn't control my desire to eat."

When Jeremy was eighteen and left home for college, he was five feet, eleven inches and 125 pounds. In college, free from his mother's control and from the limitations of his family's poverty, Jeremy rebelled against his mother by eating whatever he wanted, whenever he wanted. By the time he graduated college, he weighed almost 220 pounds. His weight continued to balloon throughout his twenties and thirties, up to 280 pounds. "I fought to lose the weight at intervals," he says. "My early training and discipline in diets and exercise helped me to rapidly lose weight, but I was never able to keep it off for more than a few months at a time."

***

In the popular book, *How to Win Friends and Influence People*, Dale Carnegie writes that, to influence someone to do something, you need to create in that person an eager want. For someone to do something—move to another part of the country, buy a new car, or lose weight and keep it off—he or she must *want* to do it.

At first thought, that might sound obvious. Of course, you have to want to do something in order to do it. But there is more to it than that. Most of us want things, but we're often not willing to do what it takes to acquire or achieve those things. So, we settle for less than what we really want, and somehow we're okay with that. We accept that life is not always going to be the way we want. Wanting something isn't enough; there must be something behind that want that makes you act to do it. And that something is called *intention*.

Habit 1 of successful weight losers is living with intention. Intention literally means the determination to act in a certain way and to be persistent in that action. If you don't *want* to successfully lose weight *to the point of changing your behavior*, it isn't going to happen; you'll regain the weight you lost, and you'll be in the never-ending cycle of lose weight, gain weight, lose weight, gain weight. Every creation happens twice: first in your head with the vision and intention you set, and second with your persistent actions that spread from that vision and intention. Persistent is the key word here, because any intention you set today must have consequential actions for the future. If you set an intention today to do something next week, how are you going to make sure that the thing you intend to do next week will get done? Responsibilities of life, as we all know, tend to get in the way. Suppose you intend today to drive from Brooklyn, New York, over the Brooklyn Bridge tomorrow to visit Manhattan, perhaps dine at Tavern on the Green in Central Park and see a Broadway show. Your intention today does not pass through time and control your action tomorrow. Tomorrow, you will have to set the same intention again to drive over the Brooklyn Bridge. So, why set an intention today about what to do tomorrow? Why not just cross your bridge when you come to it? The answer is *persistence*. Your intentions today *can* control your actions tomorrow if there is persistence in those intentions. The intentions you set must be impervious to time—even a New York minute—and to perceived obstacles. So, you don't have to cross your bridge when you come to it; you can cross your bridge today by creating the intention in your head to physically cross it tomorrow.

One of the main reasons why intention matters to be a successful weight loser is because weight loss and maintenance don't (and can't) happen accidentally. Aside from being sick with an acute illness like the flu or a chronic illness like cancer, you don't accidentally lose weight, and you certainly don't accidentally keep the weight off. You must make the decision to be a successful weight loser, and then learn and employ the required habits, with the help of environmental cues. When you live with intention, you eliminate the random approach to weight-loss maintenance in favor of the systematic and methodical one that leads to results. Research from the NWCR has shown that, when intention is behind weight-loss maintenance (which is often defined by scientists as keeping off at least 10 percent of body weight for at least one year), 21 percent of overweight people are successful weight losers.[25]

The better weight losers are at nipping any weight regain in the bud, the better the chances of it not getting out of hand and them not returning to being overweight or obese. One of the NWCR studies, published in *American Journal of Clinical Nutrition* in 2003, followed 2,258 members who regained weight to study who would reverse their weight regain and who would continue to gain weight.[26] One year after entering the NWCR, 65.7 percent gained weight. Of those individuals, only 11 percent returned to their baseline weight or below it after two years. Of the individuals who gained 1 to 3 percent of their initial body weight after one year, only 17.5 percent were able to return to their baseline weight or below it after two years. Of the individuals who gained 3 to 5 percent of their initial body weight after one year, only 14.4 percent were at their baseline weight or below it after two years. Larger weight regains reduced the chances of recovery even more. Individuals who gained the most weight after one year were the least likely to re-lose weight the following year. Conversely, those who had recovered from their weight regain had gained significantly less weight after one year than those who failed to recover. Interestingly, losing weight after regaining it affected these individuals' minds as well as their waistlines—they were less depressed compared to individuals who were unable to lose their regained weight. Although modest weight regain was common in this group (averaging 8.4 pounds) and recovery from even minor weight regain was rare, 96.4 percent of NWCR members who regained weight remained more than 10 percent below their maximum lifetime weight after two years, and they maintained an average 26.6 percent weight loss from their maximum weight.

The longer individuals have kept their weight off, the easier it is to maintain it and the less likely they are to regain the weight.[27,28] The amount of time your weight is maintained can actually predict if you'll gain weight or will continue to maintain your weight. NWCR members who have maintained their weight loss for at least two years at the time they enter the NWCR are at less risk of gaining weight one year later compared to those who have maintained their weight loss for fewer than two years. Specifically, maintaining one's weight loss for at least two years decreases the risk of subsequent weight regain by 50 percent.[29,30] If you're able to maintain your weight loss for at least two years, you'll be increasingly likely to continue maintaining it.

In one of the NWCR studies that examined this issue deeper, weight-loss durations and the habits associated with them were analyzed in 931 registry members (758 women and 173 men) who maintained an average weight loss of 62.3 pounds and had maintained at least a thirty-pound weight loss for an average of 6.8 years, with a range of two to sixty-seven years.[31] The researchers found a significant relationship between the duration of weight maintenance and the total number of weight-loss strategies used in the past year, with increasing duration associated with use of fewer strategies. Members who had kept weight off for longer said that significantly less attention and effort were required to maintain their weight. For example, individuals who had kept their weight off for longer were less likely to keep a picture of themselves in a prominent place or keep records of how much food they consumed or how much exercise they did. The duration of weight maintenance was inversely related to the effort needed to maintain weight: the longer people kept their weight off, the fewer strategies they needed to continue keeping weight off. In other words, weight maintenance got easier. The longer you persist in your intention and behave in accord with that intention, the easier it is for that behavior to "stick" and turn into a habit.

What makes one individual persist at a specific behavior while another individual doesn't? For starters, the persistent individual has a conscientious personality. One of the factors studied by the NWCR is the personality trait of conscientiousness. Conscientious individuals are efficient, organized, self-disciplined, self-controlled, goal-directed, task- and achievement-oriented, and responsible. In the most recent NWCR study, published in *Health Psychology* in 2020, conscientiousness was compared between 968 successful weight losers from the NWCR and 484 non-NWCR weight regainers.[32] The successful weight losers were found to be more conscientious than the weight regainers and scored higher on measures of order, virtue, responsibility, and industriousness. The scientists suggest that being conscientious may help individuals maintain their weight loss by improving adherence to specific behaviors.

The likelihood of you engaging in a health behavior, such as exercising or eating more fruit, is correlated with the strength of your intention to engage in the behavior. This relationship is called the Theory of Planned Behavior.[33] A behavioral intention represents your commitment to act and is itself the outcome of a combination of several variables. According to the Theory of Planned Behavior, the factors that directly influence your intention to engage in a particular behavior include your attitude toward that behavior (i.e., how favorable or unfavorable your appraisal of the behavior is), your perception of the social pressure to perform or not perform the behavior, and your perception of the amount of control you have over the behavior (i.e., how easy or difficult you perceive the behavior to be, which is strongly influenced by your past experience[34]). The more favorable your attitude toward and perception of the social pressure of the behavior and the greater your perceived behavioral control, the stronger your intention will be to perform the particular behavior. Research has shown that the factors of the Theory of Planned Behavior can actually predict health behaviors. In a review of fifty-six studies that contained fifty-eight health behavior applications of the Theory of

Planned Behavior, researchers at Université Laval in Québec, Canada, and the University of Limburg in the Netherlands found that intention remained the most important predictor of health behavior, explaining 66 percent of the variance.[35] In half of the reviewed studies, perceived behavioral control (believing that you have control over your behavior) significantly added to the prediction.

Persistence in behavior also comes from your belief about the result your effort will have. If you don't think you're going to be successful, why try at all? In 1964, psychologist Victor Vroom proposed that the strength of your tendency to act a certain way depends on the strength of your expectation of a given outcome and its attractiveness.[36] Vroom's expectancy theory is one of the most widely accepted explanations of motivation. You are motivated to exert a high level of effort when you believe (1) your effort will lead to a good performance, (2) the good performance will lead to a reward or outcome, and (3) the reward or outcome satisfies your personal goals. To adopt the habits in this book and become a successful weight loser, you must know what you believe.

All the factors of Vroom's expectancy theory, as well as the Theory of Planned Behavior, are influenced by your beliefs. It is through one's beliefs that we can learn about the unique factors that cause one person to engage in a specific behavior, yet cause another to follow a different path. In this regard, this book, and the habits contained in it, is about what you believe.

Intention not only must come from in you, it must come from the right place in you. For example, do you get pleasure and enjoyment from eating chocolate cake, or worry and guilt? Researchers in the Department of Psychology at the University of Canterbury in New Zealand wanted to find out how feelings about eating chocolate cake were related to differences in attitudes, perceived behavioral control, and intentions in relation to healthy eating and if those feelings were related to weight change.[37] Interestingly, guilt about eating chocolate cake was not a motivator for eating healthy, nor did the guilt help individuals lose weight or maintain weight loss compared to those who associated chocolate cake with celebration. The scientists discovered that those who felt guilty perceived that they had less control over their eating behavior, were less successful at losing weight over three months, and were less successful at maintaining their weight over eighteen months compared to those associating chocolate cake with enjoyment and celebration. Guilt simply doesn't work to change behavior, because it doesn't positively impact your intentions. Enjoyment and celebration are more impactful.

How do you create an eager want? By creating the conditions that are likely to cause you to want it. A gardener can't motivate a plant to grow. Rather, he seeks and implements the right combination of sunlight, nourishment, and water so that the plant "wants" to grow. How can you leverage your environment so that you want to act? If eating by yourself has created the habit of eating high-calorie, unhealthy meals, how about setting appointments to eat with others at healthy restaurants? Or calling on a friend who already eats healthy to show you how to eat healthy, too? If having a busy job prevents you from exercising, how about making a daily date with your spouse to go for an early-morning walk with you before you both leave the house for work? Find things or people who are in your current environment that support and encourage your wants. Be the gardener who makes your plant want to grow.

Becoming a successful weight loser isn't just about slimming your waistline and thighs or getting rid of your jiggly arms. It's not even about the confidence you gain from looking in the mirror. It's about conceiving to do something and then doing it, to live with purpose and intention. When you live with intention, you eliminate the random, fad-diet approach to weight loss and maintenance in favor of the systematic and methodical one that gets results. When you believe that you can accomplish anything, that is true personal freedom. You are no longer timid or scared of pursuing something, because your intention has empowered you to be bolder.

Creating the Habit

To become a successful weight loser, it's not enough to read a book about the habits of successful weight losers in hopes that you will adopt them. You must first live with the intention to form the habits of successful weight losers and then create the cues in your environment to make the habits automatic.

Habits stick when they operate outside of your consciousness. Although intentions are conscious and voluntary and habits are unconscious and automatic, they are, of course, related, as your intentions precede the practice of the actions that lead to habits. Similarly, to break your existing bad habits—which are also automatic—that thwart your weight maintenance goals, you need to remove the cues that have created those bad habits to bring your behavior under intentional control. Once you have intentional control over the bad habits, you can then set the intention to create a new, good habit. The process of intention-action-habit is a process that takes much longer than the time it takes to read this book. Living with intention is the first habit to develop, because the other behavioral actions and habits will flow from this first one.

To create the habit of living with intention, take a piece of paper and pencil and write down what you believe. Do you believe that you can lose weight and keep it off? Do you believe the effort required to do so will pay off? Will the outcome satisfy your goals? Do you believe that you must have access to a gym, a formal weight-loss program, or a personal trainer to get results? If so, how do you intend to acquire those things? Do you believe you can be a successful weight loser on your own? Do you believe that obstacles will get in your way? If so, what are those obstacles? Do you believe you have the intention and persistence to overcome those obstacles? If not, how do you think you can acquire or develop those intentions? Write all these things down on the paper. Go ahead, I'll wait.

Once you have written all the answers to the above questions, the next step to living with intention is to set goals. Goals direct your efforts, leading you to specific outcomes and achievements. When you set goals, you plant the initial seeds to set your intention—and then eventually change your behavior—in an effort to achieve them. You become more productive, focusing on the things that will get you there, and eliminating the things that won't. Goals should include the following:

Process-Oriented: People who want to lose weight and keep it off almost always focus on the pounds on the scale. The number on the scale is an outcome, and outcomes can only be controlled by focusing on the process. Putting all the eggs in the scale-means-everything basket is a great way to be disappointed if it doesn't work out. Although it's hard to lose and maintain weight without expectations, you are more likely to be a successful weight loser if you focus on the process rather than on the outcome. If you want to lose fifty pounds and stay within five pounds of that weight loss, you can have that as the end-goal, but set smaller, process-oriented goals to achieve it. It sounds cliché, but you must focus on the overall journey and the process of that journey to obtain the outcome. If you feel you have failed at reaching your goal, don't get discouraged; it likely means you didn't focus on your journey and the process to the goal, only the goal itself. Focus on the process.

Specific: Your goal should be specific rather than general. The more specific, the better. "Do your best," while a common goal used for everything from weight loss to good grades in school, is nonspecific. What does it mean to do one's best? How do you know if you have done your best? Choose a specific goal that is meaningful to you.

Measurable: If a goal cannot be measured, how do you know if it's achieved? You need to be able to measure it.

Attainable/Realistic: Your goals should be challenging, something you have to reach for, but within your reach.

Time-Bound: Goals should have a deadline to create a sense of urgency. A timeline keeps you on task.

Examples of Goals

Process-Oriented	Outcome-Oriented
Complete at least three hundred minutes of exercise this week by walking or jogging forty-five minutes every day.	Lose one hundred pounds.

Specific	Nonspecific
Eat 1,200 to 1,400 calories per day every day this week by reading nutrition labels and making decisions based on the information.	Do your best.

Measurable	Nonmeasurable
Eat three servings of vegetables and fruit per day every day this week.	Eat healthier.

Attainable/Realistic	Unattainable/Unrealistic
Lose fifty pounds in eight months and maintain a weight within five pounds of that weight loss by creating the specific habits necessary to accomplish that.	Lose fifty pounds in one month and maintain a fifty-pound weight loss for twenty years.

Time-Bound	Non-Time-Bound
Lose twenty-five pounds by December 31.	Lose twenty-five pounds.

Using these guidelines, write down your goals on a piece of paper. Make sure they are personal; they must come from within you. No one can set goals or the intention to achieve them for you. No one can coach your desire. A friend, relative, or personal trainer can try to inspire you to initiate specific actions, but you must eagerly *want* to become a successful weight loser. That want cannot come from a place of guilt about your weight or about satisfying someone else's expectations. It must come from a place deep inside of you, from your own fulfillment, from your own joy, of wanting to be more than you currently are. When you have an eager want, you have written down your specific goals, and you believe your actions will achieve those goals, you'll find the intention to act. Repeating this process—want, goal, belief—leads to living a life with intention.

***

Jeremy Kirkham's mother died morbidly obese in 2013 at age sixty, when he was just thirty-nine years old. "She had two heart attacks in two days, the second one proving fatal," he says. The ER doctor who first treated her told him that his mother's heart showed signs of weakening from untreated diabetes for over a decade. "My mother maintained a sedentary lifestyle in the last years of her life and proudly made it known that she never went to a doctor. My mother's death was the prime triggering event that led me to commit to finally conquering my weight problem once and for all. I buried my mother and made an appointment for my first ever doctor's visit on the way home from the cemetery." Despite all his yo-yo dieting and morbid obesity, Jeremy was lucky that he hadn't yet done any permanent damage to himself. "All that was left was for me to radically alter my diet and lifestyle," he says.

To lose weight, Jeremy exercised and restricted calories. "I ultimately discovered that what worked best for me was regular exercise and a plant-based diet, to which I have remained committed since the summer of 2018." To combat his sedentary occupation as an attorney, he renovated his office to include standing desks.

At 170 pounds, Jeremy has lost 110 pounds. After many years of yo-yo dieting, this time his weight loss was a straight line. He has remained within ten pounds of his current weight since reaching it in April 2019. He says that the weight loss and maintenance process was extremely difficult until he committed to a plant-based diet.

"One important thing that I learned along the way is that my commitment and drive cannot overcome my healthy appetite," he admits. "The plant-based diet helped me to bridge the gap by adding food that has a low caloric density so that I can continue to have the experience of eating a lot of food without packing on the weight."

Discovering the NWCR through an online article, he decided to join. "Through decades of dieting and failure, I thought that I had finally found a lasting positive solution, at least for myself. If the NWCR was a way to share that solution with someone who might benefit from it, I didn't want to miss a chance to help."

One of the habits Jeremy developed through this process is something he calls "flooding the zone." He explains, "If I have to attend a family or business function where I know high-calorie, tempting food will be served, I fill up on healthy food before I go. That way, the possibility of me being tempted is greatly diminished."

As a successful weight loser having overcome his mother's influence, I asked Jeremy how his mother's treatment makes him feel now. "I feel as if I served a thirty-five-year sentence for a crime I didn't commit," he says. "However insanely wrong-headed Mother was, whatever insecurities and crises within her own mind led her to treat me as she did, there is one inescapable conclusion: if she had known then what I know about nutrition today, the weakness of obesity she saw in me would have been corrected in about six months. I would have been spared the torture through which I was put, the health risks to which I was exposed, the negative social consequences of obesity, the lost opportunities, and the decades of self-loathing. Might she have instead found another worrisome flaw in me? Maybe. Maybe my nose is too big, and my eyes are too far apart. But I can more easily forgive the things about me I can't change. The weight, as something that could somehow be within my control, was an unforgivable burden that I had to shoulder."

Back at his job, Jeremy has transformed how he and others behave. "It was once the custom in the hearing room for appellants to present evidence to me by handing it to the bailiff," he says, "which I then reviewed and passed to the prosecuting attorney for her review. Now, when evidence is presented to me, I stand up to receive and review it, and then I walk it to the assistant county attorney. The assistant county attorney is now developing the practice of standing up and walking over to me to receive evidence after I review it. What was once a custom that encouraged sedentary behavior has been transformed to do the opposite. It just takes a little thought!"

When asked what advice he has for others and what he wants people to know about maintaining weight loss, Jeremy says, "It's important that as many people as possible learn that long-term weight loss is achievable, and that doing so is critical. However, restricting access to food is a sure way to failure. No matter how strong you are, your body will eventually rebel. So, find food that is low in caloric density, that will help fill you up on a regular basis. Also, exercise is very important in maintaining your health, but it puts a demand on your body that makes you want more food. You can't exercise your way out of your weight problem in the long run without also addressing your diet. Your diet is not something you do for a few months to prepare for a special occasion; it is the way you eat for life."

HABIT 1

LIVE WITH INTENTION.

HABIT 2

Control Yourself

"I VIEW MY BODY AS A PROCESS RATHER THAN AS AN OBJECT."

At the convergence of the Allegheny, Monongahela, and Ohio rivers in Pennsylvania sits the steel city of Pittsburgh, boasting more than three hundred steel-related businesses and 446 bridges. It is the home of twenty-six-year-old Emily Kilar, one of the younger members of the NWCR.

Emily was raised in a large family, literally. Both of her parents and several relatives are overweight. In middle school, Emily weighed 180 pounds. She wanted to be a cheerleader in high school.

After losing twenty pounds in one month and experiencing heart palpitations and anxiety in seventh grade, Emily was diagnosed with Graves' disease, an autoimmune disease that causes an overproduction of thyroid hormones, called hyperthyroidism. Your thyroid gland sits below your Adam's apple in your neck. It synthesizes thyroid hormone, which plays several roles, including increasing your metabolic rate. With Graves' disease, the body makes antibodies—called thyroid-stimulating immunoglobulins—that attack healthy thyroid cells, which stimulates the overproduction of thyroid hormones. The result is an accelerated metabolism and, as Emily experienced, rapid weight loss.

To treat her Graves' disease, Emily was prescribed medication to slow her thyroid function. She was also prescribed a beta blocker for her heart palpitations, which reduces cardiac output and blood pressure by causing the heart to beat slower and with less force. But there were complications. Emily's thyroid medication was too powerful, causing an *under*production of her thyroid hormones—*hypo*thyroidism—that persisted for a year and a half. And the beta blockers made physical activity difficult. She was no longer able to continue playing volleyball and going to gym class.

As a result, Emily started to gain weight. A lot. So much so that it became noticeable. Her clothes no longer fit. She wasn't enjoying daily life. Her scale read 232 pounds. "Gaining weight happened so quickly," she says. "Adjusting to my new body size was extremely difficult for my teenage brain. I felt like a prisoner in my own body. My female teenage body was larger than a grown man's. I didn't realize how large I was. I was bumping into things. I wouldn't even admit that I needed new clothes. I wore the same two pairs of pants my freshman year of high school."

She was even weight shamed by her endocrinologist. "Every time I saw the doctor, all I heard was her disappointment that I gained more weight," she remembers. She was never referred to a dietitian, instead being told how dangerous her weight gain was and to eat almonds instead of chips and soda. "I didn't even drink soda and felt extremely misunderstood," she says. She began to hide her eating, eating alone in the closet instead of in front of people. "Anxiety and depression were taking over my life," she says.

Her endocrinologist told her that her thyroid hormone level was now so low that it was as if her metabolism thought she were eating three times the number of calories that she actually was. "I was devastated," she says. Since the medication wasn't normalizing her thyroid hormone levels, her endocrinologist suggested something drastic: remove Emily's thyroid gland. Emily decided not to do the surgery, instead opting for radioactive iodine therapy, which destroys thyroid cells so that the thyroid gland cannot make thyroid hormone. When a small dose of radioactive iodine is swallowed, it is absorbed into the bloodstream and concentrated by the thyroid gland, where it begins destroying the gland's cells. As a result, Emily would be required to be on hormone replacement therapy for the rest of her life.

***

Imagine that you are sitting in an empty room at a table with a plate of cookies and are told you can have one cookie now or two cookies later. Which option would you choose? Such a scenario was used in the 1960s and 1970s by psychologist Walter Mischel, PhD, and his colleagues at Stanford University to examine the psychology of delayed gratification and self-control among preschool children.[38,39]

In the first of their series of fascinating experiments, which later became known as the Marshmallow Test, a preschool child sat at a table, on which lay five small pretzels and an opaque cake tin. Under the cake tin were five large pretzels and two animal cookies. (In other experiments, the researchers used other treats, including marshmallows, which gave the experiments their name.) The researcher explained to the child that if he left the room, the child could make him come back by eating one of the small pretzels. This was repeated with four of the five small pretzels, with the researcher leaving the room and the child eating the small pretzel to bring the researcher back into the room. Then, the researcher lifted the cake tin, revealing the bigger rewards (five large pretzels and two cookies). The researcher asked the child which of the two rewards he liked better and, after the child chose, told the child that in order for him to eat the one he liked better, he will have to sit very still in his chair and wait until the researcher came back into the room. But, if the child wanted to bring the researcher back earlier, he could do so by eating the one small pretzel left on the table. However, if the child ate the small pretzel, he couldn't eat the reward that he chose from under the cake tin. Thus, the child had a choice: he could either continue waiting for the more preferred reward until the researcher returned on his own, or he could stop waiting by eating the small pretzel to bring the researcher back into the room. If he stopped waiting, then he would receive the less favorable, but more immediately available, reward and not receive the more preferred one. Each of the thirty-two children who took part in the experiment was left waiting in the room by himself under one of four conditions: (1) with both the delayed and immediate rewards (the large pretzels and the cookies), (2) with the delayed but more preferred reward, (3) with the immediate but less preferred reward, or (4) with neither reward. In all four conditions, the small pretzel, which was the signal for summoning the researcher back into the room, was left on the table in front of the child.

What did the researchers find from this experiment? The children waited the longest time in condition 4, in which neither the delayed nor the immediate reward was available for the children's attention while they waited. In contrast, the children waited the shortest time in condition 1, when both the delayed and the immediate rewards were on the table in front of them while they waited. In other words, the children waited much longer for rewards when the rewards were absent from their view and attention than when they were present.

In a simpler version of the same experiment, each child sat in a room at a table with a plate that had one Oreo cookie in one corner of the plate and two Oreo cookies in the other corner. There was also a bell on the table. Each child was told that he or she could ring the bell after the researcher left the room to bring her back into the room and could then eat one Oreo cookie or wait until the researcher came back on her own and could then eat two Oreo cookies. Both the immediate reward (one cookie) and delayed reward (two cookies) were left in the room with the child.

In another similar experiment, Dr. Mischel and his colleagues found that when the children were waiting for the preferred but delayed reward with the reward objects in their view, delay of gratification was minimal. However, when the children engaged in fun activities to distract them while they were waiting, their ability to delay gratification was dramatically enhanced. In addition, when the children thought about the absent rewards, it was just as difficult for them to delay gratification as when the rewards were directly in their view.

From the results of his experiments, Dr. Mischel concluded that people can wait for something without frustration if they expect that they really will get the deferred larger outcome later, and, in the meantime, shift their attention elsewhere and occupy themselves with distractions.

Dr. Mischel's experiments served as a tool for studying how people go from choosing to delay gratification to actually managing to wait and resist the temptation. Diverting one's attention away from the delayed reward (while maintaining behavior directed toward its ultimate attainment) may be a key step in managing temptation. That is, learning not to think about what one is awaiting makes it easier to delay gratification, much more than does thinking about the outcome.

Although the results of the Marshmallow Test are interesting, it was what happened years after the experiments that made them famous. Many years later, Dr. Mischel and his research team decided to contact as many of the more than 550 preschoolers as they could find to compare characteristics between the now teenagers and adults who were able to delay gratification as children to those who were not. In short, the researchers discovered that the preschoolers who delayed gratification longer on the Marshmallow Test were rated as teenagers by their teachers and parents as exhibiting more self-control in frustrating situations; yielding less to temptation; being less distractible when trying to concentrate; being more intelligent, self-reliant, and confident; and more trusting of their own judgement. In addition, the preschoolers who delayed gratification longer earned much better SAT scores. The children with the longest delay times scored 210 points higher on the SAT (as teenagers more than ten years later) than the children with the shortest delay times. Even many years later, as adults, differences were still observable. Between ages twenty-five and thirty, those who had delayed gratification for longer when they were preschoolers reported that they were better able to pursue and reach long-term goals, had reached higher educational levels, and weighed less, with significantly lower body mass index. Interestingly, the researchers found that, while individuals who had lifelong low self-control did not have difficulty controlling their brains under most conditions of everyday life, they experienced problems with their behavior and brain activity when they were faced with attractive temptations.

Aside from food being the children's reward in Dr. Mischel's experiments, the Marshmallow Test clearly has implications for successful weight loss and maintenance. Being a successful weight loser requires a lot of self-control, delaying gratification now (e.g., dessert) for the more desirable reward later (e.g., a slimmer waistline, better health, enhanced self-esteem, and happiness). Unfortunately, when it comes to food, humans are rather poor at controlling themselves. We often give into temptation, allowing our emotions to control our language, our self-talk, and our behavior. If there's a free chocolate chip cookie or slice of pizza sitting on the table in front of us, many of us are likely to eat it. I know I would. We are all kids in the proverbial candy store.

People fail at weight loss—as well as other things in life— because they act in ways that reward now rather than in ways that reward later. When you have an extra ounce of energy or a few minutes of time, you'll invest that energy or time— instinctively and unconsciously—in behaving in a way that gives you immediate satisfaction. Going out to your favorite restaurant, watching a reality TV show, and scrolling through Facebook and Instagram all satisfy an immediate need and provide an immediate reward. In contrast, investments in successful weight loss don't pay off for a long time. As a consequence, we often sabotage ourselves and our happiness. Given the overwhelming availability of high-calorie, processed food in our society and the technology that steers us toward sedentary lives, you must develop strategies to distract yourself from all that attractive temptation and regulate your behavior. If you can learn to not eat the chocolate chip cookie or pizza in favor of the bigger reward—the many physical, psychological, and emotional benefits that come with keeping your weight off—you, too, will be a successful weight loser. This is exactly what the successful weight losers from the NWCR do.

Habit 2 of successful weight losers is self-control. They are aware of their actions and don't give in to temptation. Like a tourniquet to stop a bleed, most NWCR members even have a strategy in mind to implement to get back to their acceptable body weight if they regain some of their lost weight.

Self-control means voluntarily delaying a reward. If you desire the delayed outcome, you must impose the oftentimes frustrating waiting period upon yourself, like the preschoolers in Dr. Mischel's Marshmallow Test, foregoing the immediately available outcome for the sake of the delayed, but more desirable, alternative. A major problem in maintaining behaviors that enable achievement of the more desirable alternative—successful weight loss—is that the environment in which we live encourages behaviors that oppose those that predict success. The predominance of fast-food restaurants, coffee shops that sell a lot of stuff besides coffee, food-centered social gatherings, the internet that enables purchases with a finger click instead of a walk through the mall, and smartphones and social media that glue our eyes to screens and our butts to seats make it nearly impossible for people to succeed at weight loss. A key way that the NWCR members differ from typical unsuccessful dieters is that they are better able to resist temptation, control themselves, and push back against the environment. People who control themselves don't actually experience many temptations. They are not conflicted by having lots of desires that are inappropriate or out of line with their goals. In contrast, people who don't control themselves, who are unsuccessful in achieving their goals, experience many temptations.

One of the key factors of self-control is disinhibition. Disinhibition literally means not being inhibited. Some inhibition is good, because it prevents you from not giving into temptation and eating whatever and how much you want. High levels of disinhibition are bad, because it leads to risky behavior. Disinhibited eating is a failure to maintain control over eating. The opposite of disinhibited eating is dietary restraint. Multiple NWCR studies have found that increased disinhibition leads to regaining lost weight.[40-44]

How much disinhibition or dietary restraint you have is, at least partially, controlled by your brain. Brain research on obese, previously obese, and normal-weight, never-obese individuals has shown a strong link between obesity and impaired function of the brain's reward network.[45] Obesity is associated with both structural and functional alterations in brain areas related to reward anticipation, inhibition, and restraint. The good news is that you can reverse this disinhibition with weight loss. When you lose weight and keep it off, your brain activity changes compared to when you were obese. Compared to obese and normal-weight individuals, successful weight losers' brains show greater activation in the left superior frontal region, indicating greater inhibition and restraint (i.e., less disinhibition). When successful weight losers are given food, their brain reacts much like that of obese individuals—with an elevated feeling of reward—but their brain compensates with a consequently greater inhibitory control against food cues.

The Eating Inventory is a widely used measure in obesity research that has often been used to predict weight loss outcomes. Among many other questions, it includes sixteen questions that assess disinhibition (eating in response to emotional, cognitive, or social cues). There are two types of disinhibition: external disinhibition and internal disinhibition. External disinhibition refers to the tendency to eat in response to environmental (external) cues. Examples of external disinhibition include overeating when you're with someone who is overeating and eating too much at social events, where there's a lot of food. Internal disinhibition refers to the tendency to eat in response to thoughts, feelings, and emotional (internal) cues. Examples of internal disinhibition include eating to console yourself when you feel lonely and splurging on high-calorie foods while on a diet if you've eaten a food that the diet doesn't allow.

When comparing external and internal disinhibition, the latter has greater consequences. In one of the NWCR studies, published in *Obesity* in 2007, the researchers examined the effects of internal and external disinhibition on weight loss over time in 2,765 NWCR members (average age of 47.2 years) and 286 overweight men and women (average age of 40.7 years) from outside of the NWCR who were in a behavioral weight-loss treatment program.[46] For the NWCR members, higher levels of internal disinhibition predicted more weight regain a year later. In fact, each additional point on the internal disinhibition scale predicted an increase of 0.57 pound over the year. For those in the weight-loss treatment program, higher levels of internal disinhibition predicted less weight loss six and eighteen months later. External disinhibition, on the other hand, did not predict weight loss or weight regain over time in either group. The study's results suggest that the experience of eating in response to emotions or thoughts (internal disinhibition) is associated with poorer outcomes after losing weight. Another NWCR study on 5,320 members who lost an average 71.9 pounds (a whopping 30.2 percent of body weight), and kept it off an average of 5.2 years, found that higher internal disinhibition scores at entry into the registry and at one and three years later were significantly associated with poorer weight loss and faster weight regain two, four, and five years after joining the NWCR.[47] As in the other study, external disinhibition did not predict weight regain. However, individuals who had high internal disinhibition regained more weight if they also had high external disinhibition. Thus, external disinhibition may play a role in regaining weight when high internal disinhibition is present. In other words, your environment can influence your eating behavior if you have negative thoughts and feelings about food. Other studies independent of the NWCR have also found that negative thoughts and feelings (e.g., anxiety, anger, loneliness) result in dietary lapses and eating temptations.[48-52]

In one of the NWCR studies, the researchers specifically tested self-control, comparing it between NWCR members and a separate group of obese and nonobese individuals.[53] All subjects of the study were asked a series of questions about receiving a specific amount of money now or more money after a specified delay (a number of weeks, months, or years). The successful weight losers from the NWCR discounted future monetary rewards significantly less than did the group of obese and nonobese individuals. In other words, they showed an enhanced ability to delay gratification, much like the preschoolers of the Marshmallow Test who became more successful and lower-weight adults. This difference was also observed between the nonobese and obese individuals of the separate group. Other studies have found strong relationships between *a lack of* self-control—impulsivity—and obesity.[54-56] As we saw earlier, the lack of preschoolers' self-control in grabbing the pretzels, cookies, or marshmallows predicted their lack of success many years later.

Learning self-control is possible by being more conscious of your choices, monitoring yourself and your actions, and integrating the habits in this book. Most self-regulation theories consider self-monitoring an essential element of behavioral self-regulation.[57,58] One of the key behaviors that distinguishes successful weight losers from those who put the weight back on is frequent self-monitoring.[59-63]

The most common self-monitoring strategy of successful weight losers is to restrict certain foods, with 87.6 percent of NWCR registry members doing so.[64] Forty-four percent limit the quantities of food they eat and 43 percent count calories. Perhaps most importantly, they catch "slips" before they turn into larger weight regains. Interestingly, the NWCR has found that those who allow themselves more diet flexibility on holidays had greater risk of regaining weight. What sets successful weight losers apart is that they maintain a consistent eating pattern with little variety. Allowing for flexibility in the diet increases exposure to high-risk situations, creating more opportunity to lose control.

Another key self-monitoring strategy of successful weight losers is self-weighing. Although many fitness professionals advise people to "forget the scale," and claim that it's not what the scale reads, it's how your clothes fit that matters, it seems logical that if the goal is to maintain weight loss, it is important to know one's weight. If you want to be a successful businessperson, you have to know your numbers. If you want to be a successful weight loser, you also have to know your numbers. NWCR members weigh themselves regularly. In one of the summaries of their research, published in *Annual Review of Nutrition* in 2001, the NWCR reports that over 44 percent of its members weigh themselves at least once per day and 31 percent weigh themselves at least once per week.[65] A later study, based on 2,462 NWCR members, published in *Obesity* in 2007, found that 36.2 percent weigh themselves at least once per day, 42.5 percent weigh themselves at least once per week, and 21.3 percent weigh themselves less than once per week.[66] Thus, 79 percent weigh themselves at least weekly. The researchers followed up with the NWCR members a year after entry into the registry and found that individuals who increased how often they weighed themselves gained less weight (2.4 pounds) than individuals who decreased how often they weighed themselves (8.8 pounds) and individuals who weighed themselves just as often (4.0 pounds). Thus, maintaining or increasing self-weighing frequency was associated with less weight regain one year later. The study also found that individuals who decreased their self-weighing frequency were more likely to increase their percentage of caloric intake from fat, increase their disinhibition about eating, and decrease their ability to control their thoughts about food (called cognitive restraint). Even when accounting for changes in fat intake, disinhibition, and cognitive restraint, decreasing self-weighing frequency was also independently associated with greater weight regain, meaning that weighing oneself frequently is important by itself, even in the absence of other factors. Another study independent of the NWCR found that 55.1 percent of successful weight losers weighed themselves at least once per week, compared to 35.7 percent of individuals who had regained their weight, and 34.5 percent of individuals who had never been overweight.[67] Frequent self-weighing increases one's control over how much one eats and thereby helps individuals maintain their successful weight loss. If you don't weigh yourself, how do you know if you have gained or lost weight? Relying solely on how your clothes fit doesn't work.

Yet another way successful weight losers monitor themselves is by using digital health technology. A study published in *Obesity Science and Practice* in 2017 compared data tracking and smartphone usage patterns of NWCR members to individuals outside of the registry who took part in a national health survey.[68] Compared to the individuals from the external national sample, the NWCR members had 5.2 times greater odds for using any method of tracking and recording their own weight, diet, and exercise, 2.5 times greater odds for tracking these variables on a regular basis, 10 times greater odds of having smartphone apps to track or manage their health, 22.8 greater odds for using diet, food, or calorie counter apps, and 15.5 times greater odds for using an app to monitor their weight.

To control yourself, you need to become aware of what you're doing. That may seem obvious, but most of us are not aware of what we're doing. For example, when you go to see a movie, would you eat the popcorn if it were stale? According to University of Southern California psychologist Wendy Wood, PhD, you would, if you always eat popcorn at a movie theater.[69] In her experiment, ninety-eight people were seated in a movie theater and told that they were there to rate a series of movie trailers. Each study participant was given a box of popcorn upon entering the theater. Some participants received fresh popcorn, while others received stale popcorn that was popped a week before the experiment.

The participants who don't regularly eat popcorn in a movie theater ate a lot of the fresh popcorn but avoided the stale popcorn. No surprise. However, the participants who often ate popcorn at the movies ate 70 percent of the popcorn given to them, whether it was fresh or stale. When asked afterward how much they liked the popcorn, they all said that they hated the stale popcorn. But they ate it anyway.

It's hard to break habits. When experienced in the right context—in this case, a movie theater—the cues were so strong that people responded to them without thinking. They put the stale popcorn in their mouths and, even though they didn't like it, they still ate it, because, in the context of watching a movie in a movie theater, they eat popcorn. People with strong habits tend to repeat responses independently of their intentions when they are in familiar context of the behavior.

To test whether the same results would occur if eating popcorn were done differently, and therefore force the participants' behavior to be under intentional control, Dr. Wood and her colleagues repeated the experiment, except this time the participants were asked to eat the popcorn with their nondominant hand—those who were right-handed ate the popcorn with their left hand, and those who were left-handed ate the popcorn with their right hand. By throwing in this twist, the researchers were able to test whether participants with strong popcorn-eating habits would be hindered in automatically repeating their past behavior and instead would respond to the popcorn's freshness, eating only the popcorn that they liked. Interestingly, the participants who had a strong habit of eating popcorn at the movies stopped eating the stale popcorn when they had to eat it with their nondominant hand.

What can we learn from Wendy Wood's popcorn experiment? For starters, habits are inherently hidden from our conscious view. In order to create new habits to become a successful weight loser, you must be acutely aware of the habits that have kept you an unsuccessful weight loser, including those that made you fat in the first place. Once you become aware of the habits that have been keeping you where you are, you are in a power position to make a change. To stop an undesirable habit, avoid the cues that cause the unwanted behavior, and find ways to make the habit more conscious and less automatic, so that you are more mindful of the habit as you are doing the activity. For example, the easiest way to avoid the cues to buy potato chips in the supermarket is to not walk down the potato chip aisle. Step away from the aisle! Conversely, to create a desirable habit, build something into the habit to make it as automatic and independent of conscious thought as possible.

One might say that being a successful weight loser requires a bit of obsessive compulsiveness. However, you probably already have some obsessive-compulsive characteristics that you may not even be aware of. That's not the same thing as an obsessive-compulsive disorder. Obsessive-compulsive characteristics are relatively common and easily distinguished from obsessive-compulsive disorders. Research from the field of sport psychology has shown that obsessive-compulsive behaviors can actually be beneficial to athletic performance.[70-74] Given the consistency of behaviors of successful weight losers of the NWCR, obsessive-compulsive behaviors can also be beneficial to weight loss maintenance due to their ability to help you control yourself and self-regulate your behavior. Having some obsessive-compulsive behaviors is okay and is even psychologically healthy. Individuals who are more psychologically healthy may be more likely to be successful weight losers than those who fail, because they may be better able to tolerate and adjust to the environment and the pressures produced by weight suppression. The NWCR has found no evidence that maintenance of reduced body weight is associated with adverse psychological side effects.

Creating the Habit

To create the habit of controlling yourself, you need to practice. At first, this may be difficult. Think of something related to your weight-loss/weight-maintenance life that you want to change. Perhaps you want to eat fewer potato chips and more apples. When you are in the supermarket, practice bypassing the potato chip aisle, and go to the produce section instead to pick out a delicious apple. This may take some work if you are always used to walking down the potato chip aisle. Remember, to reduce or eliminate an undesirable habit, you need to do something or have a cue from your environment to bring that habit under intentional control. How about walking through the supermarket in a different pattern than you typically do? If you typically start at the front of the store and work your way to the back of the store, perhaps start at the back of the store and work your way to the front. Or, if you typically start on the left end of the store and walk up and down each aisle, perhaps start at the right end of the store and go to the produce section first, followed by walking down all of the even-numbered aisles and then walking down the odd-numbered aisles. Create a game out of grocery shopping.

Not buying potato chips at the supermarket is one thing; not eating them when you're at a social function and they are staring at you from the serving table is quite another. This is a perfect time to practice controlling yourself. Put a cue in place that makes you aware of your habit of going to the table to put food on your plate. Ask yourself, "Am I grabbing food because I am hungry or because that's the thing people do at these types of functions?" Just asking yourself this question may be enough to place the habit under intentional control.

In addition to practicing self-control to eliminate undesirable habits, you can practice self-control to create desirable habits. Perhaps you want to go to the gym to take a group exercise class. Put a cue in place that will encourage you to do that. Ask a friend to go with you, schedule an appointment to meet that friend at the gym, and tell that friend to call or text you thirty minutes before your scheduled appointment. That phone call is your cue to control yourself by getting into your car and driving to the gym.

You can practice controlling yourself to create or amplify the other habits of successful weight losers or any number of things you want to change in your life. Once you have created Habit 1, Live with Intention, practice controlling yourself to take the specific actions to reach your goals.

***

As the research from the NWCR has shown, most of us have a tipping point, that triggering event or circumstance that makes us act, that makes us do something we wouldn't otherwise do. Concerning weight loss, that triggering event is often medical. For Emily Kilar, the triggering event was the destruction of her thyroid gland from radiation therapy. "Once my thyroid was gone, I decided this was the best time to put full effort into my weight-loss journey," she says.

With her overweight family eating the typical American diet, Emily tried to pull away from those habits to lose weight. She went grocery shopping by herself. Every morning she either went for a walk or exercised to a Pilates video. She went to the gym and ran on the treadmill. "I didn't love exercise," she says. "It was kind of torturous." However, determined to lose weight, she kept at it. She lost enough weight to realize her dream of being a cheerleader in her senior year of high school.

Focusing on exercise and eating better, Emily lost sixty pounds in four years. She has since maintained her weight between 170 and 180 pounds while prioritizing her mental health. "Weight loss is all about positive mindset and consistent efforts," she says. "Both intrinsic and extrinsic motivations helped me. I wasn't going to accept my fate as being a large person."

After all the ups and downs of her weight-loss journey, she wanted to help others understand that they could accomplish what she did. She joined the NWCR, earned a bachelor's degree in dietetics, a master's degree in nutrition, and is a public health nutritionist for the Special Supplemental Nutrition Program for Women, Infants, and Children (WIC), which serves to safeguard the health of low-income women, infants, and children up to age five who are at nutritional risk by providing nutritious foods to supplement diets, information on healthy eating, and referrals to health care.

As for the habits Emily has adopted to be a successful weight loser, they reflect the habits of the NWCR. Emily's go-to physical activities are walking and yoga. "Yoga is my favorite," she says. "If exercise is not sustainable or realistic, I will never do it. I hate running!" she exclaims. Maintaining weight is harder than losing it, she says, because you can do everything to restrict calories and exercise more, but once a weight-loss goal is reached, there's no specific goal anymore. "So, why not just eat all the chips I want and sit on the couch?" she asks. Intuitive eating has been the most helpful to her, because it is realistic and focuses on feelings of hunger and fullness. Indeed, her views of food are just as important as her actual behaviors. "It's so important to accept eating decisions and cravings, honor them, and move on!" she exclaims. "Overthinking and obsessing about eating decisions crowds the mind."

Emily brings lunch to work that she prepares at home. If she buys something for lunch, she always eats healthy food. She drinks only water. She sometimes allows herself to drink alcohol in social situations which, she says, is important to her, because she used to be very strict with herself, which affected her mental health. "I believe in moderation and giving myself grace in social situations," she says.

Giving yourself grace is important. Being a successful weight loser is surely fraught with ups and downs—literally and figuratively. Your weight will go up and down and so will your emotions. Success is rarely a linear path. We tend to beat ourselves up when we fail and when we don't meet the standards we set for ourselves. Grace can go a long way to keeping you on the path (and preventing depression) as you go through your weight-loss and maintenance journey.

When I ask Emily what she wants others to know about becoming a successful weight loser, she speaks with the eloquence and perspective of someone much wiser than her years. "If someone wants to lose weight, he or she needs to know five things: First, you need to have the correct mindset. You must focus on methods that will work for you." She adds that seeking professional help is a good idea to establish a realistic plan. "I think I would have benefited from having a health professional assist me in my weight-loss journey," she says. "Establish and write down realistic short-term and long-term goals. Second, know that your body will be confused when you try to lose weight, because weight loss is not biologically normal. The body likes to store fat for times of need. You'll need to change how you have been eating and exercising. Third, eating more whole foods is nonnegotiable. Your body needs fruits, vegetables, and fiber every day. Chemicals and additives are best to be avoided. Fourth, sustainable weight loss takes time, and you need to be committed to this long term. It's important to understand a quick fix does not work. Fifth, having a support system is huge! Speak honestly with family, friends, and health care professionals about your feelings, goals, and accomplishments. I wish I had been more vocal about my mental health struggles with my doctors and family."

Throughout her successful weight-loss journey, Emily says she learned much about herself, most importantly self-control. "I learned that I could say no to things that don't serve me and I can say yes to things I'm not familiar with. I try new foods, like fruits and vegetables, instead of saying, 'No, I don't like this.' I look at food as a chance to nourish my body. My relationship with food is very logical. If something doesn't provide a nutritious benefit, I don't see much value in consuming it."

Emily continues to educate herself, reading and evaluating research about body image, which has helped her accept her body. "I view my body as a process rather than as an object," she says.

HABIT 2

CONTROL YOURSELF.

HABIT 3

Control Calories

**"I WOULD BUY MYSELF A CANDY BAR AFTER
EVERY APPOINTMENT WITH A PHYSICIAN."**

In 2009, a couple of months before her thirtieth birthday, freelance writer and research assistant Summer Yule sat in her doctor's office in Avon, Connecticut, as she was told she had stage 2A breast cancer. "My world was turned upside down," she says.

For most of Summer's life, she had been at the high end of a healthy weight, sometimes crossing over into being overweight. Introverted and uncoordinated, she was not particularly motivated to participate in group sports and was sedentary throughout her teens and twenties. "I didn't consider myself a 'fitness person,'" she admits, "and I felt at that point that I was in good enough shape that I did not need to make any changes."

Even though she wasn't active into young adulthood, she was interested in nutrition. "I ate a lot of fruits and vegetables and adopted a vegan diet during my twenties," she says. "Looking back, I don't believe this way of eating was optimal for my overall health, but I think the restrictions did ultimately help me with weight management." Since many unhealthy food options, like cakes, cupcakes, and cookies contain some eggs or dairy, her veganism took those options off the table. Instead, she stuck with whole food options like whole grains and legumes.

After her cancer diagnosis, she decided to relax her dietary restrictions and returned to eating meat as she started chemotherapy treatments, thinking that having access to a wider dietary variety would help her to maintain her weight.

With a history of low bone mineral density and iron-deficiency anemia, her change in diet alleviated those issues.

Chemotherapy dramatically altered Summer's perceptions of taste and smell. "Combined with feelings of nausea, it was extremely difficult to eat, especially for the first few days after each treatment," she says. "Thankfully, I was able to maintain my weight with the help of anti-emetic medications and trying to eat whenever I felt I could tolerate food." Her last chemotherapy treatment was at the end of 2009, after which she faced a number of painful surgeries for a mastectomy and reconstruction.

To get herself through this rough time, Summer developed a lot of bad lifestyle habits. "I would buy myself a candy bar after every appointment with a physician," she says. She was able to get away with her poor food choices because her appetite was suppressed, and she was eating very little in general. However, her lifestyle choices eventually caught up with her.

In 2011, with her perceptions of taste and smell back to full force and no longer feeling nauseous from chemotherapy, other medications, or surgery, she was enjoying food again and had a great appetite. She continued the dietary strategies that helped her maintain her weight during chemo, and she rapidly started putting on weight, tipping the scale at 195 pounds by the end of the year. "I attributed this rapid weight gain to a medication change," she says. "Looking back now, I think a number of factors caused the weight gain. So, while a change in appetite related to medication changes may have played a role in my weight gain, it was not the whole picture. Initially, I was unable to see that."

By the summer of 2012, shortly before Summer's thirty-third birthday, the largest-size clothes that she had in her closet were becoming too small. "My husband wanted to have a family photo taken, but I refused since I was so ashamed of how I looked," she says. That summer, she tripped on a curb in front of the library and twisted her ankle. It was a month before she could walk again. "That was the last straw and what I consider the event that finally spurred me to make changes," she says. During that month, Summer and her family took a trip to an amusement park, and she used an electric wheelchair since she couldn't walk comfortably. "When I looked through the photos from that trip, I was shocked at how I looked," she says. "I could barely recognize myself anymore since I had put on so much weight." The excess weight and lack of fitness had a negative impact on her quality of life. "Earlier that year, I went on a hike with my family and had to turn back because I was unable to pull myself up the rocky ledges on the trail," she says. "I had had enough and knew that the time had come to start making serious changes. Reducing my risk for future chronic diseases was a motivating factor as well." After learning she weighed 195 pounds, she stopped stepping on the scale. "My last doctor's visit revealed that I was over 40 percent body fat," she says. "It is highly likely that I was somewhere over two hundred pounds."

***

Would you eat more food from a plate or bowl simply if the plate or bowl were larger? According to many scientific studies, you would. And you wouldn't even be aware that you ate more. Research has shown that the quantity of food people consume is influenced by simple manipulations, such as plate and serving size.[75] In a study at Cornell University, people attending a

movie were given popcorn in different-sized containers. Those
served with large containers ate 45.3 percent more popcorn.[76]
The influence of the container size was so powerful that, even
when the individuals were given stale popcorn, they still ate
33.6 percent more popcorn when eating from a larger container
than from a smaller container. In case M&Ms are your snack
of choice, that, too, is subject to the size of the container
from which you're eating, even when portion size is the same
between small and large containers.[77] Even when people serve
themselves, they place more food on their plates if the plates
are bigger. What's even more interesting is that when people
are asked if they served themselves more food with the bigger
plate, they don't think they have. People are not aware of how
much they're eating. And that's a problem, because contained
in the amount of food that you're not aware you're eating are...
Wait for it...

Calories.

Calories are everywhere we turn—in the news, on food labels,
in menus, on our (larger) plates, and in our glasses and cups.
Some may even hide under your bed. We are consumed,
figuratively and literally, with calories.

Technically speaking, a calorie isn't so bad. It's rather small,
after all. One calorie is the amount of heat energy needed to
raise the temperature of one gram of water by one degree
Celsius. That's kind of esoteric, unless you plan on heating a
gram of water on your stove and measuring its energy. What's
important to understand is that when we talk about calories,
we are talking about energy. Despite the bad rap that calories
get, a calorie is neither good nor bad. It just is. It's energy. How
can energy be a bad thing?

Calories are used by nutritionists, dietitians, and food chemists to measure the amount of energy contained in the chemical bonds of the nutrients in food. Every food and beverage label includes the number of calories per serving. Because a calorie is such a small unit of energy, the unit "kilocalorie" is used to make the number more relatable. One kilocalorie equals a thousand calories. When you see a nutrition label or menu say that something has a hundred calories, it really means a hundred kilocalories, which is 100,000 calories. That number would scare a lot of people (and take up a lot more room on food labels), so food companies use kilocalories instead, writing it as Calories with a capital C. (For the purpose of simplicity and to avoid confusion, I use the term "calorie" throughout this book to mean "kilocalorie.") All those calories you eat and drink every day are used for various bodily functions in a large, complex process called... Wait for it...

Metabolism.

The word *metabolism* gets thrown around a lot, but is often a confusing subject. Metabolism is the sum of all chemical reactions inside your body. As it pertains to body weight, it is the process by which your body converts the food you eat into energy that it can use. That energy, which you learned about in high school biology class, is ATP (adenosine triphosphate). To produce ATP from food, the chemical reactions of metabolism use oxygen from the air you breathe in and produce carbon dioxide that you breathe out. (In addition to ATP and carbon dioxide, other byproducts of metabolism are water, heat, and, in the case of protein metabolism, urea.)

In 1780, French scientists Antoine Laurent Lavoisier and Pierre-Simon Laplace were the first scientists to study and quantify this process of metabolism. By measuring how much oxygen guinea pigs consumed and how much carbon dioxide they produced while sitting in a *calorimeter* (a device for measuring heat energy that is sealed off to the outside environment) and doing normal guinea pig activities, Drs. Lavoisier and Laplace could calculate, based on the chemistry of the aerobic combustion of carbohydrate and fat, their *metabolic rate*—how many calories the guinea pigs used. Pretty ingenious, huh?

The processes that control and affect metabolism are an enormously complex subject that includes the interdisciplinary fields of biology, physiology, chemistry, and physics. Adding the conditions of food intake and exercise makes the understanding of metabolism even more complex. For example, when Lavoisier and chemist Armand Séguin studied the influence of food intake and muscular work on metabolism, they discovered that resting energy metabolism increased by 50 percent due to food intake, 200 percent due to exercise, and 300 percent by combining food intake with exercise. The calories you consume every day are used either for immediate energy or stored for later use. The partitioning of calories all depends on your immediate metabolic needs.

In simple terms, when you deposit more calories than you spend, you gain weight. When you spend (withdraw) more calories than you deposit, you lose weight. Thus, your body's caloric bank account is the balance between how much you deposit and how much you spend. Successful weight loss is a permanently balanced bank account: the deposits are never more than the withdrawals, and they are often less. In order to balance the bank account permanently, the daily deposits need to be controlled because, in this particular bank account, it's much easier to make deposits than to make withdrawals. However, excess deposits are not desirable. Managing deposits every day is key to successful weight-loss maintenance.

Habit 3 of successful weight losers is controlling calories. The members of the NWCR make a lot fewer daily caloric deposits than the general population. Table 1 shows the number of calories the NWCR members consume per day from the several studies that have reported it, along with the amount of weight they lost at the time they entered the NWCR.

Table 1: Caloric Intake of Successful Weight Losers

	CALORIES PER DAY	POUNDS LOST
	1,381 [78,79]	66
	1,297 (women)	63 (women)
	1,725 (men)	78 (men)
	1,306 (women) [80]	63 (women)
	1,685 (men)	77 (men)
	1,390 [81]	69
	1,462 [82]	124
	1,400 [83]	62
	1,399 [84]	73
Average	**1,406**	79
Women	**1,302**	63
Men	**1,705**	78

As you can see from the table, the number of calories successful weight losers consume per day has remained the same across the studies over the years, from the earliest of the NWCR studies to the latest. Successful weight losers consume a low-calorie diet of about 1,400 calories per day, with women consuming about 1,300 and men consuming about 1,700 calories per day. It's possible that these successful weight losers consume more calories than this since people typically underestimate their dietary intake by 20 to 30 percent.[85] Even with this adjustment, however, the NWCR members consume less than 1,900 calories per day. By comparison, the US adult population consumes an average of 2,120 calories per day (women consume about 1,820 calories per day and men consume about 2,480 calories per day).[86,87]

Where do all these consumed calories go? Your body has a considerable requirement for energy, even at rest. Two-thirds of your energy expenditure is required for maintenance of your body's critical functions and homeostasis of its internal environment. This energy requirement, referred to as your resting metabolic rate, is about 1,300 to 1,800 calories per day, depending on body weight (the greater one's body weight, the greater the resting metabolic rate) and metabolic efficiency. To put the NWCR's daily number of calories in perspective, successful weight losers eat about equal to (and, in the cases of the heaviest individuals, slightly less than) their resting metabolic rates. In other words, they are not eating more calories than what their bodies need to maintain homeostasis. That habit is in stark contrast to that of unsuccessful weight losers who regain their weight.

This habit of controlling calories is not exclusive to the NWCR. Other research has also found that individuals who are most successful at maintaining their weight loss consume fewer daily calories, eat smaller portions, and consume fewer snacks.[88,89] The NWCR has shown that caloric intake, and an increase in caloric intake from one year to the next, are both significant predictors of weight regain after weight loss. Thus, not only is controlling caloric deposits (i.e., the *number* of calories) important, preventing the slow deposit of calories back into the bank account (i.e., the *change* in deposit behavior over time) is also important.

For this idea of controlling calories and eating less food, we must thank Luigi Cornaro, a fifteenth century Italian nobleman who adopted a calorie-restricted diet at age thirty-five to address his failing health.[90] His popular book, *Discorsi Della Vita Sobria* (*Discourses on the Sober Life*), describes his diet, which consisted of just 350 grams of food per day (about 1,500 to 1,600 calories, ironically similar to the NWCR average), including bread, egg yolk, meat, soup, and, interestingly enough, 414 milliliters (nearly three glasses) of wine. (For comparison, one slice of white bread has eighty calories and modern-day food labels are based on two thousand calories per day.) It worked. In less than a year, the diet cured him of his ailments, including gout, stomach pain, and fever, and he went on to live to 102 years old.

It wasn't until early in the twentieth century that scientific research caught up with Luigi Cornaro. In longitudinal experiments in the 1930s using rats, scientists found that rats fed 30 to 60 percent fewer calories grew at a much slower rate, and lived nearly twice as long as rats that were fed more.[91] Since then, many studies over the last eighty-five years have shown that, from rodents to primates, controlling calories extends lifespan and protects against the deterioration of biological functions, delaying or reducing the risk of many age-related diseases. And it is key to becoming a successful weight loser.

There are several ways that successful weight losers control calories. One is by limiting how often they eat out at restaurants. People who cook meals at home consume fewer calories, have better diet quality, and consume less carbohydrate and fat.[92] NWCR members average just two and a half restaurant meals per week.[93] They also shun fast food. In contrast to millions of people in the US and around the world, NWCR members rarely eat fast food, averaging less than one meal per week.[94] Those who regain weight tend to eat more fast food. The most successful weight losers actually have very little variety in their diets and don't splurge on high-calorie foods on weekends or holidays.

In addition to eating at home, successful weight losers limit how many calories they drink, especially high-caloric beverages. Most people consume a lot of unnecessary calories from beverages. Indeed, some people actually drink more calories than they eat. Sodas, smoothies, coffee drinks, and fruit juices can contribute significantly to your total daily caloric deposit and become a big obstacle to becoming a successful weight loser. A single twelve-ounce can of Coca-Cola is 140 calories, with zero of those calories being nutritious. Even diet soda still contains artificial sweeteners and acts like sugar in raising insulin level and promoting weight gain.

When asked about their beverage consumption, 41.7 percent of NWCR members said that changing what they drink is very important for losing weight and 39.6 percent said that it's very important for maintaining weight loss.[95] To become successful weight losers, they increased their consumption of water and low/no-calorie or diet beverages and reduced their consumption of regular-calorie and non-diet beverages. Only 0.9 percent drink regular-calorie soda, 0.7 percent drink mixed drinks, 0.7 percent drink hard liquor, 0.7 percent drink regular-calorie sports drinks, 0.2 percent drink low/no-calorie energy drinks, and 0 percent drink regular-calorie energy drinks or fruit juice drinks. Nearly all (91.7 percent) drink water regularly. Only 36.4 percent drink unsweetened coffee, 26.0 percent drink low/no-calorie or diet soda, 24.7 percent drink low/no-calorie or diet-sweetened coffee, 19.8 percent drink unsweetened tea, 11.5 percent drink low/no-calorie or diet-sweetened tea, and 10.8 percent drink low/no-calorie or diet-sweetened flavored water. Of those who drink low/no-calorie sweetened beverages at least once per week, 78.1 percent say they felt it helped them control or reduce the total amount of food or calories they consume.

One of the main reasons for controlling calories is because keeping weight off is even harder than losing it in the first place. There may be a few reasons for this. One of those reasons may have to do with changes to metabolism after losing weight. Research comparing resting metabolic rate before and after weight loss and between formerly obese people who have lost weight and people who have never been obese has found that weight losers burn fewer calories throughout the day than what would be expected for the new, lower body weight and compared to people of the same weight who have always been that weight.[96-100] The result is a resting metabolic rate that is, on average, 3 to 5 percent lower in the weight losers, a difference that can be explained by a low resting metabolic rate being more common among formerly obese people than among normal-weight people who have never lost weight.[101]

This "metabolic adaptation" to weight loss seems to persist for years after losing weight and even when weight is regained. A study on the contestants from TV's *The Biggest Loser* found that, despite substantial weight regain in the six years following their participation on the TV show, the contestants' resting metabolic rate remained suppressed at the same level as it was immediately after they lost all the weight on the show.[102] And it was about five hundred calories per day lower than expected based on the measured body composition changes and the increased age of the contestants.

Why does this occur? Any deviation from one's body weight—whether weight loss or weight gain—causes adjustments of caloric intake and expenditure as the body actively defends against the weight changes and attempts to return to its original weight. There may be a physiological set point or range for weight (about ten to fifteen pounds) and reducing weight below that set point or range causes physiological compensation. Thus, losing weight may create a metabolic state that favors weight regain in order to return body weight to some optimal or regulated level. Therefore, to maintain your reduced weight, you may need to eat fewer calories per pound of body weight than people who have never been overweight.

It's important to note that not all research has shown that this metabolic compensation occurs with weight loss. For example, the one study on this topic from the NWCR, which compared forty-six normal-weight individuals to forty NWCR members who had lost an average of 53.1 pounds (range = 30.0–135.2 pounds) and maintained at least a thirty-pound weight loss for an average of 9.8 years (range = 1–43 years) found that the average resting metabolic rate for the NWCR members was not significantly lower than that of the normal-weight individuals

(1,368 vs. 1,402 calories per day, respectively).[103] The researchers found no indication of increased energy efficiency (i.e., burning fewer calories per pound) in the successful weight losers. So, although some studies have shown that metabolic efficiency develops after significant weight loss that predisposes individuals to regain their weight, many people still have a normal resting metabolic rate after they lose weight.

Research has shown that an altered metabolic state could also be due to a variety of other factors, including (1) a reduced ability to burn fat, thus favoring positive fat balance and fat gain, (2) lower levels of leptin (a hormone made by fat cells that inhibits hunger and decreases fat storage), and/or (3) increased insulin sensitivity (insulin regulates glucose metabolism by triggering the transportation of glucose from your blood into cells to be used for energy).[104-106]

In addition to the possibility of your metabolism working against you and making your life difficult, your brain has its own sense of what you should weigh, no matter what you consciously believe. Your brain responds to weight loss by using powerful tools to push your weight back up to what it considers normal. If you lose a lot of weight, your brain reacts as if it were starving, and your body will burn less energy during the day in order to conserve energy. Although this was a successful survival strategy to conserve energy during the time of our early ancestors when food was scarce, it is not a good strategy in our obesogenic environment, in which high-caloric foods are in overabundance. This means that a successful weight loser—someone who does not gain the weight back—must forever be vigilant in eating fewer calories and being more physically active than someone of the same normal weight who has always been that weight.

To examine this issue further, a NWCR study compared weight management during the holidays between 167 NWCR members and a separate sample of ninety normal-weight individuals.[107] Holidays present a time that challenges intention and caloric control. Between company holiday parties and family vacations, it's easy to let habits slip, not go to the gym, and eat more than a few gingerbread cookies. Perhaps anticipating the forthcoming temptations, the successful weight losers were very intentional. They were more likely than the normal-weight individuals to have plans to be extremely strict in maintaining their usual dietary and exercise routines during the holidays. They paid greater attention before and after the holidays to their weight and eating habits, such as daily self-weighing, and exhibited more weight control behaviors, including stimulus control techniques such as eating at one place in the home. They were more physically active and ate breakfast more often than the normal-weight individuals. They even ate less fast food. While 32.3 percent of normal-weight individuals avoided all fast food before the holidays and 35.6 percent avoided it after the holidays, 53.9 percent of successful weight losers avoided fast food before, and 50.3 percent avoided it after. However, despite practicing more extreme weight control behaviors to manage their weight over the holidays, the successful weight losers, who had lost an average of seventy-seven pounds and maintained at least a thirty-pound weight loss for six years, still had greater difficulty than the normal-weight individuals in controlling their weight: 38.9 percent gained weight during the holidays, while only 16.7 percent of normal-weight individuals did, and 51.2 percent kept their weight stable within a couple of pounds, compared to 74.4 percent of the normal-weight individuals. Successful weight losers who gained weight over the holidays were far less likely to lose the weight over the next month (and to return to their preholiday weight) than were normal-weight individuals, who can get away with a lot more (e.g., eat more fast food, exercise less).

This doesn't mean that you don't have any control over how much you weigh. The successful weight losers of the NWCR are absolute proof of that. Your choices still matter. Your willpower matters. Your intention matters. Research has shown that none of the physiological or metabolic factors related to weight loss seem to be major influencers of weight regain and that differences in behavior are stronger predictors of weight regain than differences in physiology or metabolism. The people whose stories are woven through this book are proof that you do have control over your weight.

Whatever the specific compensatory biological mechanisms that may exist after losing weight, one thing is clear: when you lose weight, you need to eat fewer calories per pound of body weight than people who have never been obese to maintain your reduced weight. And to do that requires controlling calories.

Creating the Habit

There are several ways to create the habit of controlling calories:

1) Eat from a smaller plate or bowl. Since forming new habits is all about creating contextual cues that make your actions automatic, even the seemingly insignificant environmental cue of a smaller plate can have significant consequences on controlling calories, as research has shown. If you always eat from a small plate, your brain will associate "food" with "small

plate" and you'll eat less food than if you always or often eat from a large plate. Buy smaller plates and bowls so you don't have the option of filling up a larger plate.

2) Limit how often you eat out at restaurants. Although it's easy to eat out while you're running errands, on your way home with your kids from their after-school activities, or while at your job, doing so causes you to eat more. Eat at home as much as possible. This may take some planning. Pack a lunch to bring with you to your job instead of eating out. Plan your meals for each day, or even for the entire week. Reserve dinner for "family time." Set up environmental cues to make eating at home a habit.

3) Count calories. When you go grocery shopping, read the nutrition labels to check the number of calories per serving and how many servings there are in the item. See if you can guess how many calories there are in the items you want to buy. Make a game out of it. By giving yourself a reason to look at the nutrition label, you're more likely to do it and to create the habit over time. When you prepare your meals at home, keep track of how many calories you eat. Use a calorie-counting app like MyFitnessPal to input what you eat. Set a specific and measurable goal concerning the number of calories. Remember that successful weight losers consume an average of 1,400 calories per day. If you measure it, you can manage it.

4) Follow a consistent meal schedule. If the craziness of daily life gets in the way and you don't think you can do this on your own, set an alarm for specific mealtimes. If you eat at consistent times every day, you're less likely to overconsume calories whenever food is around. Use an alarm as your cue to eat. If this sounds familiar, it is. It's an example of classical

conditioning, which you may have learned in high school or college psychology class. When you pair a conditioned, neutral stimulus, like an alarm, with an unconditioned, biologically potent stimulus, like food, the conditioned stimulus will, over time, elicit a conditioned response, like salivation, that is similar to the response elicited by the unconditioned stimulus. In other words, the sound of an alarm, when paired with eating a meal, will, over time, condition you to only eat at specific times of the day.

5) Eat slowly. By slowing down the rate at which you eat, you're more likely to stop when (or even before) you are full. Set a timer to help you create this habit. Pick a reasonable amount of time, perhaps fifteen or twenty minutes for an average-size meal. Don't finish eating until the time has expired.

6) Drink only water. If you can't give up coffee, that's okay, but stay away from soda, fruit juices, sports and energy drinks, and anything from Starbucks. A water bottle can serve as a physical cue to drink water. Bring a water bottle with you in your car and keep it at your desk at work. If you fill up on water, you won't have room in your stomach for something else.

***

To lose weight, Summer Yule maintained a strict diet, consuming 1,200 to 1,500 calories per day, along with initiating lifestyle changes. "I think I am like many people in that I do not like to be hungry," she says. "I had to be creative to figure out new ways to compose low-calorie but satisfying meals." At her lowest weight, Summer was 125 pounds. "It was nice to get to see the changes in my body and the numbers going down on the scale. Shopping for a whole new wardrobe was fun, too!"

At age forty, Summer currently weighs 130 to 135 pounds and has kept off sixty-five to seventy pounds for seven years. After her weight-loss journey, Summer went back to school to become a registered dietitian and learned the importance of individualized nutrition advice. "Specific strategies that work for me may not be what is best for someone else, so feel free to tweak what you see is working for others to fit your own life," she recommends. She owns and manages SummerYule.com, a free recipe resource for adults aged thirty or older who want to lose at least twenty pounds. She joined the NWCR because she wanted to help others by contributing to the data on successful weight losers. "Maintaining the consistency needed for healthy weight management can be challenging at times, but it is not impossible," she says.

Although she no longer has a specific calorie target she aims for, Summer is very in tune with how many calories she needs, and averages 2,000 to 2,500 calories per day to maintain her weight. As she did when losing weight, she still tracks her food on the MyFitnessPal app for accountability. "I consistently lose weight averaging under 1,900 calories," she says, "and there's a good chance I'll gain weight if I start regularly consuming over 2,000 to 2,500 calories. I don't sweat it if I have some days that are over or under this range; it's what I am doing consistently that counts." Most of her meals are rich in protein (meat, poultry, eggs, fish, and dairy) and non-starchy vegetables. "Over the years, I have learned that prioritizing protein, fiber, and fluid helps me to create meals that support both satiety and healthy weight management," she says. For snacks, she prefers fruit, plain yogurt, and air-popped popcorn. She doesn't subscribe to a particular way of eating, such as low-carb or vegetarianism, but she eats mostly whole foods with limited added sugar and refined grains. While she doesn't officially restrict any foods or drinks, she rarely, if ever, consumes sugar-sweetened beverages.

Aside from diet, physical activity is an essential part of her weight maintenance. She typically averages one hour of exercise per day, six days per week. Day seven is errands day, during which she is on her feet a large portion of the day. "My most common physical activity routine is a 10K run or walk three days per week and a workout video the other three days," she says. "I mix these up with seasonal activities, like cross-country skiing, sledding, and hiking."

Summer says that one of the most challenging things about weight maintenance is that it can be a bit boring. "Something I've learned about myself is that I enjoy variety. Mixing things up with new workouts and different healthy recipes keeps me motivated to maintain my lifestyle."

HABIT 3

CONTROL CALORIES.

HABIT 4

Eat a Low-Fat, High-Carbohydrate Diet

**"I CAME HOME WEIGHING EXACTLY THE SAME AS WHEN I
LEFT, EVEN WITH A GLASS OR TWO OF WINE EVERY DAY."**

Retired physics and chemistry teacher from St. Peter, Minnesota, Diann Marten sits at a café in France with her French friend and eats dessert. She takes a few bites and shares the rest with her friend. She does this every day for the twelve days she's on vacation. Before leaving on the trip, her friend asked her what she wanted to do while in France. "Eat dessert every day," Diann replied.

Diann started overeating when she was five years old, when her baby sister was born. "I could capture the attention of my brothers or my mom by asking for food," she says. By third grade, Diann was seriously overweight. Kids teased her. Her mother took her to the doctor, who proclaimed her healthy and told her not to worry. Her mother put her on a diet anyway. To escape the food restriction at home, Diann ran over to her grandparents' house to eat. "Those were the first days of my binging behavior," she says. "I remember my grandfather giving me a disgusted look as I ate multiple servings of cookies and ice cream."

Despite her rebellious binging at her grandparents' house, her mother's diet worked. By the time she entered middle school, she was normal weight, although she still felt overweight because she was taller and bigger than her friends. "I took it upon myself to diet, sometimes eating only an egg a day," she says. (Extreme dieting like this can be dangerous and cause health issues.) At five feet, nine inches, she got down to 119 pounds, with a below-normal body mass index of 17.6. "Then I made friends with alcohol and marijuana," she says. Those friends, combined with partying at college and more binging, brought her weight up to 180 pounds.

Years later, married with two sons, Diann weighed 225 pounds. "I was a successful teacher, working on my master's degree, but I wasn't happy," she says. "My husband had serious anger issues and my binging was the worst it had ever been." She got divorced and became a single mom.

A new boyfriend encouraged her to lose weight. "He told me, 'If you really want to lose weight, you'll have to exercise enough to work up a sweat,'" she says. "So, I started running. I ran 10K races, ate sensibly, and got down to 169 pounds." She completed her master's degree, was offered a teaching job with better pay and benefits, and moved far enough away that she and her boyfriend broke up.

At her new job, she met the love of her life and married him after nine months of dating. "We celebrated every day with big dinners that included lots of bread and wine," she says. Her weight gradually increased to 253 pounds, the highest it had ever been. Her knees hurt and she had plantar fasciitis, which made it difficult to walk. "I had everything I ever wanted in life, but I was severely depressed," she says. "I hid it well, never missed a day of teaching, but, often, I was in bed by eight o'clock. I tried a diet now and then, but nothing worked."

Then she saw a photo of her taken at her son's prom. "I cried, because I looked so terrible," she says. "I knew then that I needed help and that I couldn't do it alone." She researched weight-loss programs and decided on Weight Watchers. "I was hesitant because I had tried Weight Watchers once before and really didn't believe it would work for me," she says. "But

I forced myself to go to a meeting, thinking that if I didn't like it, at least I tried."

***

The many proponents of low-carb diets would have the public believe that carbohydrate is poison. The gurus say that carbohydrate is the reason for the obesity epidemic and that people should avoid it like the plague. What an irony it is, then, that carbohydrate, in the form of the sugar glucose, is the body's preferred and immediate source of energy, with carbohydrate metabolism evolving long before fat metabolism came along.

It may be surprising (and almost certainly thwart their marketing) for those weight-loss gurus to discover that a high-carb, low-fat diet is the rule rather than the exception for the successful weight losers of the NWCR. You read that right—successful weight losers eat a high-carb diet.

Habit 4 of successful weight losers is eating a low-fat, high-carb diet. Table 2 shows the percentage of carbohydrate, fat, and protein the NWCR members consume, from the several studies that have reported it.

Table 2: Macronutrient Consumption of Successful Weight Losers

	% FAT	% CARBOHYDRATE	% PROTEIN
	24 (women) [108]	56	20
	24 (men)	56	20
	24 [109]	56	19
	23 [110]	58	19
	26 [111]	55	19
	24 [112]	56	19
	29 [113]	49	22
Average	25	55	20

As you can see from the table, NWCR members eat a low-fat, high-carbohydrate diet. They consume an average of 25 percent of their calories from fat, 55 percent from carbohydrate, and 20 percent from protein, with no difference in the macronutrient percentages between women and men. Age also doesn't make a difference in the macronutrient composition of the diet, as young adults (eighteen to thirty-five years old) and older adults (thirty-six to fifty years old) consume a similar percentage of calories from fat (as well as from alcohol, sugar-sweetened beverages, and total calories).[114]

Historically, fat has taken a lot of the blame for making people fat. Indeed, the data from the NWCR and other studies have shown that the amount of dietary fat and an increase in the percentage of calories from fat from one year to the next are both significant predictors of weight regain. However, while it's easy to think that if you eat fat, you'll get fat, fat itself doesn't make you fat. The main reason for a low-fat diet—and the presumed reason why the NWCR members control their fat intake—is because of fat's high caloric density rather than because it's fat *per se*. At nine calories per gram, fat provides a concentrated calorie source to give you energy. Fat is more than twice as calorically dense as carbohydrate and protein, both of which have four calories per gram.

Fat is actually a very important part of your diet. You can blame your brain. Your brain is an expensive organ to maintain. It's like your body's Ferrari—it needs a lot of energy, and fat contains a lot of energy. Perhaps the most significant evolutionary change in the modern human was growth of the brain, from 850 to 1,200 cubic centimeters as *Homo erectus* (between 1.5 million and 130,000 years ago) to 1,350 to 1,400 cubic centimeters as *Homo sapiens* (first showing up 130,000 years ago). Humans expend a much larger share of their resting energy budget on brain metabolism than do other primates or non-primate mammals. Where do we get the energy to support our metabolically expensive brains? From high-energy fat. Research on the diets of primates shows that the high cost of a large human brain is supported by diets that are rich in fat. Greater brain size also appears to have consequences for human body composition, particularly when we are young. Human infants have more body fat than do the infants of other mammals, which enables human brains to grow by having a ready supply of stored energy. Interestingly, when dietary fat is not readily available, human infants and toddlers preserve their body fat by stunting their body's linear growth and even increase the amount of fat they store, so the brain has enough for itself. From an evolutionary perspective, the increased consumption of fat—and thus the energy that comes with it—appears to have been necessary for promoting brain growth in humans. Fat also helps to produce hormones, is an important component of cell membranes, contributes to nerve function, and carries the fat-soluble vitamins A, D, E, and K into your bloodstream.

Although there are successful weight losers who consume a greater percentage of calories from fat and a lesser percentage from carbohydrate (e.g., individuals who have lost weight with bariatric surgery[115]), controlling the amount of fat in the diet is the more robust strategy of the NWCR to control total calories and defend against a growing waistline. Research independent of the NWCR has also found that the most successful weight losers reduce the percentage of calories from fat in their diets.[116-118] Those who consume cheese, butter, high-fat snacks, fried foods, and desserts less than once per week are more successful at long-term weight control.[119]

In the early 2000s, the fat content of the NWCR members' diet increased and the carbohydrate content of their diet decreased compared to earlier years. At that time, low-carb diets were becoming all the rage, with people pushing away the pasta and potatoes in favor of more fat and protein. The decrease in carbohydrate content of the diet seems to have come from a decrease in "bad carbs," like processed foods with added sugar, since, also during that time, NWCR members increased their consumption of vegetables to nearly four servings per day and increased their consumption of fiber from vegetables, fruit, and beans.[120] The opposite habit—an increase in dietary sweets—is a significant predictor of weight regain.[121]

The percentage of NWCR members consuming a low-carbohydrate diet (less than 90 grams, which is less than 25 percent of daily calories) increased from 5.9 percent in 1995 to 7.6 percent in 2001 to 17.1 percent in 2003, although it still remains low for successful weight losers, despite the media's attention on low-carbohydrate diets. Even with the increasing percentage of NWCR members consuming a low-carbohydrate diet, the fat content of the diet still remains far below the national average. Hardly anyone in the NWCR is consuming a very low-carbohydrate or ketogenic diet. The word "ketogenic" doesn't even exist in any of the NWCR's published studies.

This slight shift in the macronutrient composition of the NWCR members' diet came with consequences. When weight fluctuations were examined after one year, in light of the change in macronutrient composition, the increased percentage of calories from fat and decreased percentage of calories from carbohydrate were significantly related to weight regain. In other words, the lower-carb approach isn't working in the long term. This is a robust finding of the NWCR: weight regainers decrease their carb intake and increase their fat intake, whereas maintainers keep their fat intake consistently low. NWCR members who consume less than 24 percent of their daily calories from carbohydrate maintain their weight loss for less time and are less physically active than members who consume a high-carbohydrate diet.[122]

While interesting, it's little surprise that low-carbohydrate dieters exercise less than high-carbohydrate dieters. With a low-carbohydrate diet, it becomes very difficult to exercise a lot since carbohydrate is the muscles' preferred exercise fuel. Since the members of the NWCR are not asked why they consume a high-carbohydrate diet, it can only be speculated, but is likely due to the fact that they exercise a lot. Carbohydrate is vital for exercise. Muscle biopsy research since the 1960s has shown that exercise requiring cardiovascular endurance is strongly influenced by the amount of carbohydrate stored in skeletal muscles (called glycogen), with muscle glycogen depletion becoming the decisive factor limiting prolonged moderate- to high-intensity exercise. That muscles prefer carbohydrate as a fuel is fundamental to exercise metabolism, even research examining supplementation with carbohydrate *during* exercise has shown that fatigue can be delayed.[123]

To find out why muscles prefer carbohydrate, we have to go all the way back to the time life on Earth began. A long time ago, before you and I were born, the atmosphere of primitive Earth was thought to have been made up of hydrogen and contained little or no oxygen. So, the earliest organisms on Earth had to develop an anaerobic (non-oxygen-using) way of producing energy. Since carbohydrate can be broken down without oxygen—which distinguishes it from fat, which can be broken down only in the presence of oxygen—organisms relied on carbohydrate. Millions of years later, carbohydrate is still your muscles' fuel of choice.

When your carbohydrate fuel tank is low, your body doesn't perform well, and exercise, especially of a high intensity, becomes laborious. Brain function is also impaired by a lack of carbohydrate. If you don't have enough carbs, you literally can't think straight, and your reasoning skills diminish. In order to exercise at a high intensity, prevent hypoglycemia (low blood sugar), refuel your muscles, and strengthen your immune system, you need to eat enough carbs. Your body's store of carbohydrate (as glycogen in your muscles and liver) is relatively limited and can be acutely manipulated on a daily basis by your dietary intake or even by a single workout.

One NWCR study compared low-carbohydrate weight losers (e.g., those who used Atkins diet, South Beach diet, or another low-carb diet) to all other NWCR members who enrolled in the registry between 1998 and 2001 (the time when the Atkins diet and other low-carbohydrate diets were becoming popular).[124] Only 10.8 percent said they lost weight with a low-carbohydrate diet. At the time they entered the NWCR, the low-carb weight losers lost less weight than the non-low-carb weight losers (60.7 pounds vs. 70.6 pounds, respectively) and had kept their weight off for less time than the non-low-carb weight losers. Their diet was 9.5 percent carbohydrate and 64.0 percent fat (compared to 48.2 percent carbohydrate and 30.9 percent fat for the non-low-carb weight losers). Three years later, their diet had changed to 16.9 percent carbohydrate and 58.8 percent fat (the non-low-carb weight losers' diets had not changed). As had been shown in earlier research, the low-carb weight losers were much less physically active than the non-low-carb weight losers (burning 1,595 calories per week at registry entry, and 1,119 calories per week three years later vs. burning 2,542 calories per week at entry, and 2,246 calories per week three years later, respectively), however, they did not gain significantly more weight over the three years compared to the non-low-carb weight losers. (Low-carb weight losers gained 8.4 pounds after one year, 9.9 pounds after two years, and 14.3 pounds after three years; non-low-carb weight losers gained 5.1 pounds after one year, 8.8 pounds after two years, and 10.3 pounds after three years.) Other research independent of the NWCR on a random sample of weight losers has shown that low-carb dieters experience greater weight regain compared to non-low-carb dieters six to twelve months after starting their diet.[125] Since the low-carb dieters of the NWCR were already successful weight losers when they entered the registry, it is possible, albeit not the norm, to be a successful weight loser on a low-carb diet in the presence of other self-regulating behaviors.

Since there are three macronutrients, we can't forget about protein amid all this talk of fat and carbohydrate. Like an army of construction workers amid a building's scaffolding, protein is used for construction inside your body. The protein you eat is broken down into amino acids, the metaphorical bricks that are used to repair and maintain muscle mass, build new functional proteins and cells in response to specific stimuli, like exercise (e.g., mitochondria, enzymes, red blood cells, and antibodies), and build transport proteins that move molecules from one place to another (e.g., albumin, which transports fatty acids to your muscles and liver for oxidation when your blood sugar is low). Protein also makes you feel fuller, and helps control appetite. If you lack protein in your diet, not only are you likely to feel hungry more often, you're more likely to experience a decrease in muscle mass, suppressed immune system, increased risk of injury, and chronic fatigue. People at risk of insufficient protein intake include those on a very low-calorie or vegetarian or vegan diet. (Low-calorie diets put *all* nutrients at risk for being insufficient, and plant proteins are less well digested than animal proteins.) Diets that contain 0.4 gram per pound of body weight per day are effective for weight and fat loss when reducing calories to lose weight, while higher-protein diets that contain 0.5 to 0.7 gram per pound of body weight per day, and include at least 25 to 30 grams of protein per meal, provide improvements in appetite, body-weight management, and reduction in risk factors for cardiovascular and metabolic diseases.

Although the emphasis of so-called "low-carb" diets is on carbohydrate, it is primarily the relatively high-protein content of the diet that is responsible for the success that people have with such diets. That was the conclusion of scientists at the Nutrition and Toxicology Research Institute in the Netherlands, when they compared body weight and percent body fat (as well as many other variables) of 132 individuals who were randomly assigned one of four diets for twelve months: (1) low carbohydrate/high protein, (2) low carbohydrate/normal protein, (3) normal carbohydrate/high protein, and (4) normal carbohydrate/normal protein.[126] By manipulating the carbohydrate and protein contents of the diets, the scientists sought to find out whether it is the lower carbohydrate or the higher protein content of the diet that influences weight loss and maintenance. After the subjects consumed the diet for two weeks, the total calories of the four diets were reduced to 33 percent for the next three months to induce weight loss. For the next nine months after that, total calories were increased to 67 percent that of the first two weeks to maintain weight. After both the three-month weight-loss phase and the nine-month weight-maintenance phase, the amount of physical activity the subjects did had not changed, nor did it differ between groups. Here's what the macronutrient composition of the four diets looked like, with the subjects' body weight and percent body fat at the end of each phase:

	LOW CARB HIGH PROTEIN	LOW CARB NORMAL PROTEIN	NORMAL CARB HIGH PROTEIN	NORMAL CARB NORMAL PROTEIN
Phase 1 (2 weeks)				
% Carb/Protein/Fat	25/20/55	25/10/65	50/20/30	50/10/40
Phase 2 (3 months)				
% Carb/Protein/Fat	5/60/35	5/30/65	35/60/5	35/30/35
Phase 3 (9 months)				
% Carb/Protein/Fat	25/30/45	25/15/60	45/30/25	45/15/40
Phase 1 (2 weeks)				
Body Weight (lbs.)	238	236	233	232
% Body Fat	41.5	45.4	45.9	45.2
Phase 2 (3 months)				
Body Weight (lbs.)	206	209	203	208
% Body Fat	35.3	40.7	39.9	41.2
Phase 3 (9 months)				
Body Weight (lbs.)	212	215	207	214
% Body Fat	36.6	41.7	40.7	42.1

As you can see in the table, body weight and percent body fat decreased during the three-month weight-loss phase with all four diets. When calories were increased over the next nine months during the weight maintenance phase, the subjects regained some weight. There was a significant difference in the amount of weight loss between the high-protein and normal protein diets (average of 31 pounds vs. 25.5 pounds), but not between the low-carb and normal-carb diets (average of 29.5 pounds vs. 27 pounds). This was also the case after twelve months. Weight loss and weight maintenance depend on the high-protein, not on the low-carb, component of the diet. The fat content of the diets also had no effect on weight loss or weight maintenance. The scientists suggest that increasing the protein content of the diet while reducing calories may cause a greater feeling of fullness (i.e., satiety), which assists weight loss and maintenance. Research from the NWCR has shown that people who consume less protein are more likely to regain weight, compared to those who consume more protein.[127]

Manipulating macronutrients seems to be a fun exercise for scientists, as well as for the general public of dieters. What would happen to total calories of the diet if one macronutrient were increased by 1 percent while another macronutrient was decreased by 1 percent? That was the question posed by researchers at the University of Illinois, Urbana-Champaign.[128] Using data from years of calorie and macronutrient compositions of diets from the National Health and Nutrition Examination Survey (NHANES), a well-known research program conducted by the National Center for Health Statistics to assess the health and nutritional status of adults and children in the United States, the researchers found that substituting protein or carbohydrate for fat and substituting protein for carbohydrate all cause daily calories to decrease, with the largest effect coming from substituting protein for fat. Specifically, increasing the percentage of calories from protein by just 1 percent while decreasing the percentage of calories from fat by just 1 percent—a 1 percent protein-for-fat exchange—caused total daily calories to decrease by 64, 69, and 70 calories for normal-weight, overweight, and obese men, and 42, 45, and 49 calories for normal-weight, overweight, and obese women, respectively. When it comes to reducing calories, protein is kind of special: exchanging it for fat (and, to a lesser degree, for carbohydrate) makes a big difference.

One way to ensure your macronutrients are balanced to provide optimal energy for life's daily activities and to support your weight-loss success is to be consistent with your diet. The members of the NWCR who maintain the same diet across the week and throughout the year are more likely to maintain their weight loss over the following year than members who diet more strictly only on weekdays and/or during non-holiday periods.[129] Although variety has been called the spice of life, it's not the spice of successful weight losers. They limit variety in their diets, avoiding the weekend and holiday splurges and treats, probably because it's more difficult to control calories and macronutrient percentages when eating a large variety of foods each week. If you eat the same thing (or similar things) every week, it's much easier to maintain specific percentages of fat, carbs, and protein than if you're eating completely different meals every week. One study that compared diet variety between 2,237 NWCR members and recent weight losers who had not yet become successful weight losers found that the NWCR members consumed less variety from low-fat-dense food groups than the recent weight losers.[130] The largest difference in food group variety between the NWCR members and the recent weight losers was found in the food group from the top of the Food Guide Pyramid: fats, oils, and sweets, with NWCR members having less variety than recent weight losers. Although overall dietary variety is low in NWCR members, they consume more variety in nutrient-dense and low-fat-dense foods (i.e., the *bottom* of the Food Guide Pyramid) than in other food groups. In other words, successful weight losers are not wasting calories on foods and beverages that don't provide nutrition (e.g., fast-food restaurants, Starbucks, desserts, etc.). The researchers found that the variety consumed among all food groups was positively correlated to caloric intake—the more variety, the more calories consumed.

To model your diet after the NWCR, consume about 55 percent carbohydrate, 25 percent fat, and 20 percent protein. These percentages don't have to be exact; you ultimately need to find the macronutrient composition that works for you for the rest of your life. To support your level of physical activity, eat less carbohydrate at times when you are less physically active, and eat more carbohydrate at times when you are more physically active. If you reduce the percentage of carbohydrate, make up the difference with protein rather than with fat. Remember that with every gram of fat you eat or drink, you're consuming more than twice the number of calories you consume with carbohydrate and protein. Eating a low-fat, high-carbohydrate diet doesn't mean eating a huge plate of pasta at every dinner or eating lots of chocolate chip cookies. It means eating healthy carbohydrate, like fruits, vegetables, and whole grains. That's the habit of the successful weight losers.

Creating the Habit

There are several ways to create the habit of eating a low-fat, high-carbohydrate diet:

1) Plan your meals each week. Be diligent about this, otherwise the specifics of what you eat can get out of hand. Planning can prevent that from happening.

2) Every time you go to the supermarket, fill up your shopping cart with greens, fruits, and vegetables before putting anything else in your cart. Create in your mind the association of "supermarket" with "greens, fruits, and vegetables." For supermarket items that are typically high in fat, choose the low-fat options. Read the nutrition labels. If it's too difficult to place kale in your shopping cart instead of potato chips, have someone else go grocery shopping for you. If you don't have processed carbs and fatty foods in your shopping cart, they won't be in your home. If processed carbs and fatty foods are not in your home, you can't eat them. Out of sight, out of mind will work after a while.

3) Create cues in your home to eat more healthy carbohydrate and less fat. Keep a fruit bowl on the dining room table or island in your kitchen. Set a morning fruit alarm to eat fruit before you eat anything else.

4) Consult a registered dietitian or qualified nutritionist to create a meal plan for you. Following a professional's advice can eliminate the guesswork of you having to figure it out on your own.

5) Include a high-protein food at each meal. Add an egg to your breakfast oatmeal, turkey or tuna to your lunch salad, and salmon to your dinner.

6) Keep a food journal. For a few weeks to a few months, write down what you eat at every meal. Although it may seem like a pain to write everything in a journal, it will make you aware of what you currently eat and will show you where to make changes. For example, after reviewing what you wrote, you may discover that your diet has been higher in fat or lower in protein than what is optimal, and you'll be alerted to make a change in one or more macronutrients. After a while, you'll no longer need to write down what you eat, as consuming the specific foods that will help you achieve your goals becomes a habit.

Remember, for a behavior to become a habit, it must become automatic. If you repeatedly practice these strategies, the behaviors will eventually become automatic.

**

After her first Weight Watchers meeting in 2008 at age fifty, Diann Marten realized she had found a place where she could get help and be inspired. "I sat in my car after the meeting and sobbed uncontrollably with relief, because I knew that I had found what I needed," she says. In addition to Weight Watchers, she listened to a podcast called *Inside Out Weight Loss*, which helped her work through her food issues. By 2011, Diann had lost 72 pounds to reach her goal weight of 181 pounds. At one of the Weight Watchers' meetings, she heard about the NWCR and decided to join. "My weight had been such an issue for so long, and I wanted to help others understand that if I can lose and maintain it, they can, too."

In 2016, her weight crept back up to around 210, which she again lost, and has hovered around 193 pounds ever since. She has kept off sixty pounds for nine years. "I'm still working on mindful eating," she says. "At times I overeat, because I'm stressed or bored or because the food is there, but I don't remember the last time I binged."

Diann's knee pain and plantar fasciitis are gone. She plays tennis four hours per week and takes an intense yoga class at least once per week, which keeps her strong so she can keep up with her grandsons.

"There were hard times with weight loss, times when I plateaued or didn't feel like tracking my food," she says. "Those were the times when I needed my Weight Watchers group or the podcast the most. There were also really easy times when everything was working beautifully. Now, most of the time, it's pretty easy. It's still hard when I'm stressed or when I get down on myself. I learned that it's important to slow down and enjoy my food. I try to find joy in each day, and part of that joy is eating wonderful, healthy foods. I learned that I can eat! I had so much guilt around food before I found a podcast that helped me work through my food issues."

When Diann's weight increases, she logs her food to kickstart a loss. Nighttime eating is sometimes still an issue. "I'm trying to develop the habit of having a small dinner and either nothing or a small, healthy snack before bed," she says. She eats lots of fruits and vegetables and makes those her go-to foods if she feels a need to munch when she's not really hungry. She pays attention to her food and makes her meals attractive. She often uses a smaller plate or bowl. "I try to look for opportunities, not obstacles, so if I'm at a buffet, I search out great-looking fruits or veggies and good, lean proteins," she says. "I indulge and I'm determined not to feel guilty about it."

When asked what advice she has for others who want to become successful weight losers, Diann says, "You need to tell yourself how great you are, and never talk badly to yourself. If you fail, you're learning. Any diet can work, but you must focus on living it. It's easy to stay on a diet for a week, but for long-term change, pick a plan that you can live with and one that will help you change your habits for good. And find the support of a trusted friend or group."

What about that twelve-day trip to France during which Diann indulged on daily dessert with her friend? "I came home weighing exactly the same as when I left, even with a glass or two of wine every day!" she says.

HABIT 4

EAT A LOW-FAT, HIGH-CARBOHYDRATE DIET.

HABIT 5

Eat Breakfast

**"IT WAS LIKE A BOBBY FLAY-STYLE THROWDOWN, AND
I IMPRESSED THE HELL OUT OF MY HUSBAND."**

In Foster City, California, thirty-eight-year-old educator Brenda Trosin takes a shot of alcohol and mounts the elliptical machine for her workout. At 267 pounds, it's often painful for her to exercise. She works out at home because she doesn't want to be seen in public.

Growing up with a healthy weight, Brenda gained the "Freshman Fifteen" in college and continued to add eight to ten pounds per year for another decade. As her weight continued to noticeably increase year after year, she felt awkward mentoring her students in basic goal-setting principles. "If my students wanted to improve their reading skills, I preached time on task," she says. "This lesson is true for weight loss as well, and I was fully neglecting that part of my life.

As she got older, her weight became too much to carry. "I was struggling with basic tasks, like sleeping, and I was always physically tired," she says. "I received emails from my health insurance company, saying that I was eligible for bariatric surgery and inviting me to several orientations. It seemed quite wrong to modify an organ permanently to accommodate a lifetime of bad behaviors. I was very aware that I made myself fat. I owned my own mess. I did this to myself."

Outwardly, Brenda had an amazing life: a great husband, a wonderful career, and a community of solid friendships. "But, internally, I had some work to do to clean up my head," she says. "Slowly, I began to think that if I made myself fat, I might be able to make myself fit, too."

It took Brenda a few months to figure out how to start, what to implement, and where to find helpful resources. Working for a large public library system with millions of items in its collection, she had access to unlimited information. "I started studying about nutrition, reading personal weight-loss stories for inspiration, identifying my bad habits, and trying to understand the impetus of my fatness," she says. As she did her research, she discovered the NWCR, which provided behavior-based data.

Thinking she was too fat for most traditional fitness activities, Brenda decided to get an elliptical machine for her home. "I started with fifteen to twenty minutes of physical activity each day," she says. "I logged every workout on a chart. My husband purchased the equipment for me, so I was committed to log thirty days of workouts to show my appreciation."

After reaching her first thirty-day goal and seeing some improvements in her mobility, Brenda decided to keep going. After a few more months, she committed to doing 365 workouts in 365 days. (She missed only three or four days due to illness and travel during that first year.) With daily exercise now a habit, she began to address her nutrition. "During the first few months, I would implement a new behavior every few weeks, master that one, and add another one," she says. "I meal prepped. I packed my lunches. I included one cheat meal per week. I weighed myself every day. I bought a Fitbit to track steps, downloaded the MyFitnessPal app to my phone to count calories, and started tracking everything. I learned to shop smarter, cook healthier, and embrace healthy living habits."

***

Breakfast is my favorite meal. Ever since I was a kid, I have loved sugar cereals, pancakes, waffles, scrambled eggs, and hash browns; I could eat those foods all day. I often reminisce about going to International House of Pancakes (IHOP) restaurant on Sunday mornings as a kid to be treated to chocolate chip pancakes with boysenberry syrup and whipped cream, with a side of hash browns and scrambled eggs. Good times.

Although it's not a good idea as adults to keep eating those foods for breakfast, and makes it more difficult to be a successful weight loser, it turns out that your mother (and her mother, and her mother) was right, after all—breakfast really is the most important meal of the day. Few other adages have better weathered the test of time.

Habit 5 of successful weight losers is eating breakfast. In the largest of the NWCR studies on this issue, breakfast-eating behaviors were studied in 2,959 registry members (79.5 percent women, 20.5 percent men).[131] Seventy-eight percent eat breakfast every day, while only 4 percent never eat breakfast. These successful weight losers lost an average of 71.3 pounds (women lost 70.2 pounds and men lost 75.9 pounds) and maintained the NWCR-required minimum weight loss of thirty pounds for an average of six years. Of those who eat breakfast, 29.6 percent always eat cereal, 30.1 percent usually or often eat cereal, 20.6 percent sometimes eat cereal, and 19.7 percent rarely or never eat cereal. Also, 31.4 percent always eat fruit for breakfast, 24.2 percent usually or often eat fruit, 23.6 percent sometimes eat fruit, and 20.8 percent rarely or never eat fruit. Although nearly 80 percent of NWCR members eat breakfast, the researchers found no difference between breakfast eaters and non-breakfast eaters in the amount of weight lost (70.4 vs. 74.8 pounds, respectively) or in the duration of weight-loss maintenance (7.9 vs. 7.7 years, respectively). So, it's possible to be a successful weight loser without eating breakfast; however, skipping breakfast is not the norm among the successful weight losers of the NWCR. Eating breakfast every day is also common among other successful weight losers: the NWCR's sister registry in Portugal (Portuguese Weight Control Registry) has found that daily breakfast is one of their members' most common strategies.[132]

Breakfast often takes a back seat or is forgotten altogether as people pay much more attention to its mid- and late-day counterparts of lunch and dinner. Most social events that include food are organized and planned around lunch and dinner; few social events include breakfast. Between 1965 and 1991, the proportion of US adults skipping breakfast increased from 14 percent to 25 percent,[133] in part because of lack of time and a desire to control body weight. Skipping breakfast may seem logical as a weight maintenance strategy since controlling calories is one of the most important habits of successful weight losers. If you eat two meals per day instead of three, how could that not be a good idea?

Well, it's not. Research has shown that the exact opposite is the case—skipping breakfast is actually associated with consuming more total daily calories.[134] Skipping breakfast makes you hungry and therefore more likely to eat more later in the day to compensate. Breakfast-skippers also tend to weigh more than breakfast eaters, and obese individuals are more likely to skip breakfast. A study at the University of California, Berkeley, that examined the relationship between breakfast type, body mass index, and caloric intake using data from the Third National Health and Nutrition Examination Survey (NHANES III, a large, population-based study conducted in the US from 1988 to 1994) found that people who skip breakfast have a higher body mass index, and people who eat cereal (cooked or ready-to-eat) or quick breads for breakfast have a significantly lower body mass index than people who eat other types of breakfast (e.g., meat and eggs).[135] The scientists concluded, "It is clear from these and other data that skipping breakfast does not lead to attaining or maintaining a healthy weight." This population-based study agrees with the successful weight-loss behavior of the NWCR, as 78 percent of members eat breakfast every day and, for 80 percent, that breakfast, at least sometimes, includes cereal.

In another study on calorie consumption at different times of the day, scientists at the University of Murcia in Spain discovered that individuals who consumed a greater percentage of their daily calories at breakfast and skipped breakfast less often lost more weight more quickly than did those who consumed a greater percentage of their daily calories later in the day and were breakfast-skippers.[136] Another study at Tel Aviv University in Israel also found that a high-calorie breakfast results in greater weight loss than a high-calorie dinner.[137] Scientists placed ninety-three overweight and obese women on two diets containing identical macronutrient content and composition equaling 1,400 calories for twelve weeks. The only difference was that one diet emphasized a big breakfast (50 percent of daily calories) and a small dinner (14 percent of daily calories) and the other diet emphasized a big dinner and a small breakfast by reversing the percentages. After twelve weeks, the women on the high-calorie breakfast lost nearly two and a half times more weight than those on the high-calorie dinner (nineteen vs. eight pounds, respectively). Waist circumference and body mass index also decreased more with the high-calorie breakfast than with the high-calorie dinner.

To see whether the macronutrient composition of breakfast influenced weight regain after losing weight, the scientists at Tel Aviv University placed 193 overweight and obese men and women on two diets for thirty-two weeks that differed in breakfast: a low-calorie, low-carbohydrate breakfast (300 calories; 10 grams of carbohydrate; 30 grams of protein) and a high-calorie, high-carbohydrate (and high-protein) breakfast (600 calories; 60 grams of carbohydrate; 45 grams of protein).[138] Lunch and dinner were planned so that total daily calories were the same between diets. After the first sixteen weeks, both groups of individuals lost similar amounts of weight (six to seven pounds). However, after thirty-two weeks, the high-calorie/high-carb breakfast eaters lost an additional three pounds, while the low-calorie/low-carb breakfast eaters regained five pounds. Thus, the high-calorie/high-carb breakfast eaters were more successful weight losers on two accounts—they not only maintained their lost weight, they continued to lose weight. When the scientists compared factors related to hunger (e.g., satiety, cravings, and ghrelin, a hormone in the stomach that increases hunger) between the diets, they discovered that satiety was significantly higher and hunger and ghrelin were significantly lower in the high-calorie/high-carb breakfast eaters, suggesting that a high-calorie/high-carb (and high-protein) breakfast may be a more sustainable weight maintenance strategy.

So, no matter how busy you are in the morning to get your day started, skipping breakfast is not a good idea. Normal-weight and underweight individuals more evenly distribute their caloric intakes throughout the day. Eating breakfast is important for several reasons. When you first get out of bed in the morning, your blood glucose is on the low side of normal. Your body needs energy for the day's activities. Since it has been many hours since your last meal, you need to break the fast, literally. The macronutrients you eat at breakfast will be used for their important jobs—carbohydrate will be used to replenish your blood glucose from your overnight fast to provide immediate fuel for your cells and to store muscle glycogen for later use; protein will be used to maintain the structural integrity of your cells and tissues and to transport nutrients in your blood; and fat will be used to provide energy, absorb fat-soluble vitamins, and maintain your body's temperature. Because you are in a metabolically needy state when you get out of bed, all those calories from carbohydrate, protein, and fat that you eat at breakfast will be used to fulfill your body's metabolic demands. Skipping breakfast only serves to deny your body the fuel it needs.

Creating the Habit

Having the intention to eat breakfast every day and telling yourself to eat breakfast every day is not enough to eat breakfast every day. To create the habit, you must create the right environment. Add repeated situational cues to your morning routine so that you eat breakfast every day. After a while, eating breakfast every day will become automatic as your brain associates the specific cues with breakfast. There are several ways to create the habit of eating breakfast every day:

1) Make breakfast a family event. Although mornings can be busy with getting ready for work and getting kids ready for

school, breakfast is a great opportunity for family to meet together before starting the day. Sit down with your family at the kitchen table to eat breakfast every day with them. Families meetings at the table is a strong cue to engage in the behavior of eating breakfast. If everyone else is doing it, you don't want to feel left out.

2) Set the kitchen or dining room table for tomorrow morning's breakfast before going to bed. Put out the plates, the silverware, the glasses, and even the fancy cloth napkins. Make breakfast an event you look forward to.

3) Prepare breakfast the night before. Instead of sitting on the couch in the evening while watching reality TV, prepare breakfast for tomorrow morning. Make overnight oatmeal that you can reheat in the microwave in the morning or eat it right out of the refrigerator. Place a banana on the kitchen table so you see it when you walk into the kitchen. Hard boil some eggs for the week so you can easily grab an egg each morning. Focus your breakfast on carbohydrate and protein by placing those items in your line of sight.

4) Be hungry in the morning, both literally and figuratively. Don't have late-night snacks after dinner so you will literally be hungry when you wake up and encouraged to eat breakfast and start your day, hungry to live an exceptional life.

5) Set a special alarm on your smartphone that you will associate with eating breakfast, perhaps your favorite inspirational song, or a song that reminds you of breakfast, like Deep Blue Something's *Breakfast at Tiffany's* or Melissa Steel's *Kisses for Breakfast*.

***

Once Brenda Trosin started to lose a significant amount of weight, she decided to work with a fitness trainer at the gym. "I was still very uncomfortable being in public and trying something new," she says. "I am not athletic by any means, so it was a challenge for me to overcome my own mental limitations. However, everyone was so kind and supportive that I did my best to focus on that energy. As a kid who failed physical education class in the sixth grade due to attendance issues, it felt wonderful to participate in sporting activities."

One of Brenda's friends encouraged her to train for an all-women's 5K run in San Francisco. She weighed about two hundred pounds. "I was shocked to see that my fitness was decent enough to jog three miles," she says. "I got hooked on running pretty quickly after that first race." She transitioned from daily workouts on the elliptical machine to running "the mean streets of California," as she puts it, with two- to four-mile runs before work each morning. Before the end of the year, she was training for a half-marathon, which she completed in 2014. "I was the chubbiest girl in the race," she says, "but I placed well, given my total lack of experience. I found true joy in running, and I loved the community of runners in the Bay Area. Running is great therapy, so that became my best practice."

Now forty-five years old and 185 pounds, Brenda no longer takes a shot of alcohol before her workouts to numb the pain. "Those initial sessions during the first month were incredibly painful for my knees and back," she says. While she doesn't recommend that approach to others, she says that when talking fitness with her trainers and fit friends, "there are two topics that they often overlook concerning overweight people: pain management is an essential part of a weight-loss program and compression garments are our best friends."

All told, Brenda lost ninety pounds in two years, dropping her pants size from 26 to size 12. She currently lives near Orlando, Florida, and works for a publishing company as a financial resource administrator. Her weight is up slightly from the low 170s she weighed when she was running over thirty miles per week to train for a half-marathon. Even though Brenda is already a successful weight loser, having maintained nearly all her weight loss for more than five years, she's not done. "I felt really proud once I hit that critical five-year milestone," she says, "but I have a strong desire to lose more. I still dream of losing a full hundred pounds and mostly maintaining it. Everyone loves observing a project with visible progress."

Brenda's weight loss didn't come without some side effects, both to her clothes and her friends. "There were a few unexpected outcomes of this effort," she says. "I got creative with clothes for about two years because I could not afford to replace my entire wardrobe multiple times as I shrunk. I welcomed gently used clothes from my friends. I shopped secondhand consignment shops in affluent zip codes. I bought pants with ties. I found a good tailor. I also needed to replace all my shoes and get my jewelry resized. Some of my friendships were strained, and I even lost some casual friends along the way. With women, there always tends to be some subtle weight-based interactions. Once I quietly disrupted the pecking order of fatness within my circle, it changed the group dynamics."

Brenda admits that maintaining her weight has been different than losing it. "Maintenance is much harder because no one really cares," she says. "There is a very specific shift that happens for a fat-to-fit person, and it gets lonely at times when in maintenance mode. It's a lifelong commitment and an ongoing struggle."

To stay on track, Brenda has created many habits to maintain her weight. She prepares her meals days in advance. She eats breakfast. She stays hydrated. She embraces counting calories. She works out with friends. "These days, I do fewer thousand-calorie brunches," she says. "I prefer walk-and-talks with my girlfriends instead, or we get together for longer training sessions on the turf."

She also sets up several methods of accountability. She removes barriers. She exercises every day on a consistent schedule, from five to six thirty in the mornings Monday through Friday and eight to ten o'clock in the morning on weekends. "I used to tease that I was training for the Chubby Olympics," she says. "Now, I train daily at a fantastic gym with amazing trainers and friends. If I'm having an off day, I still go to the gym to run on the treadmill. I adapt. I modify. I overcome. If my knees are unhappy that day, I switch to the elliptical machine. If that still hurts, I try the bike. Usually, I can work out the pains in a few minutes of moderate movement."

A few years ago, Brenda learned that she will eventually need to have heart valve surgery. She currently takes medication and gets tested by her cardiologist every three to six months. Because of her heart condition, she monitors her heart rate to stay within safe guidelines and is required to be supervised while exercising. "Once I understood the seriousness of my heart condition, I had to shift my thinking from improving my running performance to learning to love running less competitively," she says. "Now, I obsessively watch all the major marathons around the world and follow [marathon world record holder] Eliud Kipchoge for that running rush, but I will forever be restricted to running on a treadmill at a reasonable pace under observation. I miss running on the streets, but I am grateful to have a few more miles ahead of me with my underperforming heart. I am also trying to learn to love weightlifting, and I take group step and core classes at the gym. I have learned that I am resilient."

Brenda sets many goals, writes them down, and celebrates them. In the beginning of her journey, she had incentive goals. "If I did ninety workouts in ninety days, I might treat myself to a new workout outfit," she says. Now, to maintain her weight, she always has a weight-loss goal, a fitness goal, a vanity goal, a running goal, and a fun activity goal. "I want to lose twenty more pounds," she says. "I want to deadlift 160 pounds. I want to shop at White House Black Market. I want to run the Golden Gate Bridge. I want to jump on a trampoline. Some goals might take a year to reach, so it helps to have other, smaller goals."

When asked what advice she has for others, Brenda says, "Find people and activities that bring you joy. Be brave. Tackle new challenges. Find a fitness mentor and mentor someone else. Those relationships help to keep you engaged and energized."

Brenda's weight-loss and maintenance journey has been nothing short of transformative. She has found a confidence she didn't have before. "Overall, I can do some amazing shit!" Brenda exclaims. "We recently bought a large safe for our house that weighs over three hundred pounds. I confidently told my husband that I was good for my half of the lift if he could knock out his half. It was like a [celebrity chef] Bobby Flay-style throwdown, and I impressed the hell out of my husband."

HABIT 5

EAT BREAKFAST.

HABIT 6

Exercise (a Lot) Every Day

"THERE'S A BIG PAYOFF AS I LOOK DOWN FROM A RIDGE OR A SUMMIT TO THE MESAS BELOW OR ACROSS THE UNDULATING RIDGES OF MOUNTAINS."

Above the Arctic Circle in northern Alaska sit the Arrigetch Peaks, a cluster of rugged granite spires in the Endicott Mountains in the seven hundred-mile, mostly uninhabited Brooks Mountain Range, which is believed to be about 126 million years old. The name *Arrigetch* in the Inupiat language means "fingers of the outstretched hand." Fifty-seven-year-old Jamie Ash looks out over the expansive tundra, admiring its peaking fall colors. She trained seven months for this hike.

Back home among the Sangre de Cristo Mountains in the north-central region of New Mexico, Jamie colors interior plaster using imported pigments to make a wall finish unique to northern New Mexico. She owns Handmade Plaster Pigments in the small town of Taos, which is named after the Taos Pueblo, one of the oldest continuously inhabited communities in the United States. Jamie has been living in Taos since 1985.

As an eighteen-year-old preparing to go to college, Jamie weighed 165 pounds. "I'm five feet, two and a half inches, so that made me a pretty round person," she says. "In 1979, I was an outlier." Most of her peers were a lot smaller than her. Not wanting to be so self-conscious about her body, she tried to lose weight, getting down to 135 pounds over eight weeks through exercising and eating only 900 calories per day. She got new clothes and felt attractive. Once she got to college, however, she stopped exercising and took advantage of the unlimited amount of food in the dining hall. The weight came back within two months.

When she was forty-three years old and 172 pounds, Jamie tried to lose weight again. "I knew I had gained weight since I could no longer button the top of my pants," she says. "My mother had been big, maybe two hundred pounds. When I saw 172 on the scale, I could see two hundred not far away, and I was horrified at that possible trajectory." Jamie joined a gym, started walking on a treadmill, and stopped eating sugar. She got down to the mid-150s. "I stopped trying to lose weight, but didn't think about maintaining," she says. Exercise slowly dropped away, dessert slowly came back and, within six months, so did the pounds.

When she was fifty-three, Jamie was looking for a vacation within a day's drive of Taos. During yearly trips to the Oregon Coast, she had flown over Utah and was awed by its red rock formations. "Each time I saw the land morph from green and brown to red, I thought about going back," she says. Never much of an exerciser or an outdoors person, she planned a hiking trip to Utah anyway.

***

In a review of the data from the National Health and Nutrition Examination Survey (NHANES), scientists at Stanford University's School of Medicine compared obesity, physical activity, and caloric intake in US adults from 1988 to 2010.[139] They found a significant association between the level of physical activity in the population—but not daily caloric intake—and the increases in body mass index and waist circumference. The proportion of adults who did not exercise increased dramatically from 1988 to 2010—19.1 percent to 51.7 percent among women, and 11.4 percent to 43.5 percent among men. Finding no evidence that average daily caloric intake had increased over that time period, despite a continued upward swing in obesity, the scientists' claimed that their findings do not support the popular notion that the rise in obesity in the US is primarily a result of consuming more daily calories. It's not a coincidence that two-thirds of the US adult population is overweight or obese and less than one-fifth of the population exercises on a regular basis.

Yet, many popular weight-loss plans emphasize diet more than exercise. We are told to eat this, not that. However, emphasizing diet over exercise misses an important point—cutting calories and eating a more nutritious diet does not make you fitter and doesn't do much to reset your metabolism. Nutrition doesn't give your muscles or your cardiovascular system a stimulus to which to adapt. Only exercise can provide that stimulus, sculpting your body and making you fitter and healthier. And because you must eat enough to maintain your resting metabolic rate (around 1,300 to 1,500 calories per day) so you can continue to live, caloric restriction is limited (you can't cut your calories to only 100 per day, after all). By contrast, exercise is virtually unlimited. It's hard to overdose on exercise.

One of the major reasons why exercise is the main driver of metabolic control and thus of successful weight maintenance is because of the potent effect exercise has on your muscles—specifically, the mitochondria deep inside your muscles, which are the microscopic factories responsible for aerobic metabolism. Mitochondria are full of enzymes—the factory workers—that catalyze the many chemical reactions of metabolism. Exercise stimulates the synthesis of mitochondria through a sophisticated process called mitochondrial biogenesis, making you a better fat-burning (and carbohydrate-burning) machine.

The link between an increase in mitochondrial enzyme activity and an increase in mitochondria's capacity to consume oxygen, first made in 1967 in the muscles of rats, has provided much insight into the ability of skeletal muscles to adapt. The increase in mitochondria steers your muscles' fuel use toward a greater reliance on fat at the same exercise intensity, which is one of the hallmark adaptations to aerobic exercise. In essence, exercise resets your metabolism, stimulating fat mobilization and oxidation and creating the necessary conditions that direct the calories you eat into fulfilling specific metabolic demands.

Not only does exercise positively alter your metabolism and burn more calories than anything else you do during the day, it also means you spend less time sitting on your butt, doing calorie-storing things like watching television. People who watch TV are not exercising. Watching TV is a particularly bad habit if you want to be a successful weight loser. In fact, it is so detrimental to becoming a successful weight loser, and minimizing TV viewing is such a notable finding of the NWCR, that I almost added it as an additional habit of successful weight losers. People who increase the amount of television they watch, and decrease the amount of exercise they do, are at particularly high risk for weight gain. In a NWCR study published in *Obesity Research* in 2006, researchers discovered that 63.5 percent of NWCR members watch less than ten hours of TV per week, and 38.5 percent watch less than five hours per week. Only 12.5 percent watch more than twenty-one hours of TV per week.[140] These findings are in stark contrast to the typical TV viewing behavior of American adults, who spend an average of twenty-eight hours per week watching TV.[141] The NWCR has shown that the more TV people watch, the less they exercise. People who spend a high percentage of hours watching TV engage in less total, moderate-, and heavy-intensity weekly exercise and consume a greater percentage of their total daily calories from fat (people tend to eat more high-fat snacks while watching TV). Moreover, the amount of TV viewing and an increase in amount of TV viewing from one year to the next are both significant predictors of weight regain.

When you exercise, you are also more likely to form and stick to *other* habits that make becoming a successful weight loser more likely. For example, individuals who exercise more have greater control over their diets than individuals who exercise less, including lower fat consumption and greater cognitive restraint.[142]

And that leads us to Habit 6 of successful weight losers—exercising a lot every day. Indeed, the amount of exercise that the NWCR members do is one of their most notable habits. The members of the NWCR are more physically active and burn more calories than the general population, and even more than those enrolled in behavioral weight-loss programs.[143] Most NWCR members—89.6 percent of women and 85.3 percent of men—exercise as part of their weight-loss and weight-maintenance strategy. Table 3 shows the number of calories the NWCR members burn per week during physical activity, from the several studies that have reported it, along with the amount of weight they lost at the time they entered the NWCR.

Table 3—Caloric Expenditure of Successful Weight Losers

	Calories Per Week	Pounds Lost
	2,832 [144]	69
	2,829 [145]	66
	2,985 [146]	124
	2,545 (women) [147,148]	63 (women)
	3,293 (men)	78 (men)
	2,542 [149]	71
	2,621 [150]	71
	2,521 [151]	73
Average	**2,722**	79
Women	**2,545**	63
Men	**3,293**	78

As you can see from the table, NWCR members burn a lot of calories exercising, far more than what is considered the minimum amount needed by the general public to prevent weight gain and to reduce obesity-associated risk factors for chronic disease. (Reputable organizations, like the American College of Sports Medicine, recommend 150 to 250 minutes of exercise—equaling about 1,200 to 2,000 calories—per week.[152]) The number of calories successful weight losers burn per week has remained the same across the studies over the years, from the earliest of the NWCR studies to the latest. Successful weight losers burn about 2,700 calories per week, with one study that separated the women and men in their analysis reporting that women burn about 2,500 and men burn about 3,300 calories per week.

Despite these averages, there is a lot of variability in how much exercise these successful weight losers engage in. A quarter of NWCR members burn fewer than a thousand calories per week, which suggests that there may be some individuals who can maintain their weight loss with less exercise. However, most of these successful weight losers exercise a lot: 72 percent burn more than two thousand calories per week, and 35 percent burn more than three thousand calories per week.[153,154] To put this in perspective, walking or running one mile burns about 110 calories, give or take, depending on factors like body weight and aerobic economy. This means that these successful weight losers burn the equivalent of walking or running about twenty-four miles per week, with women burning the equivalent of twenty-three miles per week and men burning the equivalent of thirty miles per week. In one of the NWCR studies, which included 3,683 members, calories burned during high-intensity exercise accounted for 34 percent of the total calories burned per week for both men and women.[155] When it comes to the amount and intensity of exercise, these successful weight losers don't mess around!

In addition to the caloric expenditure data in Table 3, another study compared the number of minutes (rather than the number of calories) of sustained moderate-to-vigorous intensity exercise between twenty-six NWCR members, thirty-four overweight individuals whose body mass index (BMI) was matched to that of the NWCR members, and thirty normal-weight individuals who were never obese. The NWCR members exercised at moderate-to-vigorous intensity for an average of 290 minutes per week (69.2 percent exercised at moderate-to-vigorous intensity for at least 150 minutes per week and 30.8 percent for at least 300 minutes per week), while overweight individuals exercised at moderate-to-vigorous intensity for an average of just 134 minutes per week, and normal-weight individuals for an average of 181 minutes per week.[156] Thus, the successful weight losers spent significantly more time each week exercising at moderate-to-vigorous intensities than their overweight counterparts and were even more physically active than their normal-weight counterparts who had never been overweight.

The finding of successful weight losers being more physically active than people who were never overweight isn't exclusive to the members of the NWCR. In a study on 237 individuals from outside of the NWCR, scientists compared the amount and intensity of exercise of successful female weight losers to individuals who had never been overweight.[157] The weight losers once had a BMI of at least 25, were of normal weight (with a BMI between 18.5 and 25) at the time of the study, had lost and kept off at least 10 percent of their maximum body weight for at least five years, and were within ten pounds of their lost weight for at least two years prior to the study. Conversely, the normal-weight individuals were never overweight and always had a BMI between 18.5 and 25. Their weight also was stable, being within ten pounds of their weight for at least two years prior to the study. The successful weight losers were very successful, reducing their weight from an average of 199.8 pounds to 132.7 pounds, and maintaining at least 10 percent weight loss for more than fourteen years. What went into this incredible amount and longevity of weight loss? The scientists discovered that the successful weight losers spent more total time each day being physically active compared to the individuals who had never been overweight

(58.6 minutes vs. 52.1 minutes), largely because they spent more time doing high-intensity exercise (24.4 minutes vs. 16.9 minutes, respectively). The majority of never-overweight individuals exercised thirty to sixty minutes per day, whereas a greater percentage of successful weight losers exercised more than sixty minutes per day.

Why do successful weight losers exercise so much? Partly because it takes a lot of exercise to prevent a return to previous weight, and partly because exercise has become a habit of this population. Ninety-two percent of NWCR members exercise at home, 40.3 percent exercise regularly with a friend, and 31.3 percent exercise in a group.[158] Walking, running, cycling, weightlifting, aerobics classes, and stair climbing are the most common physical activities. Walking is the most popular, with 76.6 percent of NWCR members doing so as their preferred mode of exercise. Those walkers average more than 11,000 steps per day.[159] Weight training has become more popular over the years, with 37.0 percent of men and 36.6 percent of women who enrolled in the registry from 2001 to 2004 doing it, compared to 25.3 of men and 22.9 percent of women who enrolled from 1993 to 1996.[160] All these data have led the founders of the NWCR to conclude that the optimal amount of exercise to maintain weight loss is about one hour per day or, in terms of caloric expenditure, 2,500 to 3,000 calories per week.[161]

Although diet usually gets more attention in conversations on weight loss and maintenance, very few successful weight losers in the NWCR use diet alone to lose weight. Only 9 percent of these successful weight losers, who were a whopping ten BMI units lower than their pre-weight-loss BMI at the time they entered the NWCR (decreasing from 35 to 25 kg/m^2), said they maintained their weight-loss (which averaged sixty-six pounds for five and a half years) without regular exercise.[162] It seems that only some successful weight losers can maintain their weight without much exercise. Among these people are those who lose weight through bariatric surgery. Surgical weight losers are much less physically active than nonsurgical weight losers, burning only half as many calories per week (1,504 vs. 2,985 calories per week, respectively).[163] (Surgical weight losers engage in different behaviors to maintain their lost weight than the rest of the NWCR. In addition to exercising much less and consuming less carbohydrate and more fat, they eat fast food more frequently and eat breakfast less frequently than nonsurgical weight losers.[164]) While changes to your nutritional habits—most crucial of which is how many calories you consume every day—have the bigger impact on getting your weight off, exercise has the bigger impact on keeping it off, and making you a successful weight loser.

In the days of "clean eating" and low-carb, vegan, paleo, gluten-free, keto, dairy-free, juice-cleanse diets, it's become trendy to claim that diet is everything. Indeed, most fitness trainers claim that physical appearance and body weight are 80 percent nutrition and 20 percent exercise, and that "abs are made in the kitchen." However, there is no scientific evidence to back up that claim. Exactly how much of a person's physique is due to nutrition, how much is due to exercise, and how much is due to genetics is difficult to determine. (Research on identical twins raised apart in different environments has shown that genetics has a large influence on body weight.[165,166]) It's presumptuous to think that the specific foods you eat are more important to your cosmetics, fitness, and health than are exercise and genetics. I'm pretty sure I didn't get my sculpted legs from eating kale salads; I got them from running six days per week for thirty-six years. And so it is for other physically active people as well. Athletes, bodybuilders, and dancers all do a considerable amount of physical training to look and perform the way they do. The sculpted legs of runners and upper bodies of fitness magazine models didn't get that way just by eating fruits and vegetables. If we take two people, and one eats perfectly clean, with a nutrient-dense diet and no processed foods, but doesn't exercise much, and the other works out in the gym every day, but has a mediocre diet with the occasional chocolate chip cookie, who is going to look better and be fitter? Obviously, the latter.

A decrease in physical activity is a major reason why people gain weight. Think of your high school's star quarterback who has a big belly at middle age. How many people at age thirty or forty or fifty weigh the same as they did in high school? The NWCR has shown that individuals who regain weight within one year show marked decreases in physical activity of more than eight hundred calories per week, with no change in overall calorie intake.[167,168] That means that weight losers are regaining their weight not because they start eating more, but because they start exercising less. This is a major finding of the NWCR—a large part of regaining weight after losing it is due to the inability to maintain exercise habits for the long term.

One NWCR study found a significant relationship between the amount of exercise and the amount of weight loss maintained, with individuals in the highest quartile of exercise maintaining a nine-pound greater weight loss than those in the lowest quartile of exercise.[169] A later study on 3,591 successful weight losers who enrolled in the NWCR from 1993 to 2004 (2,723 women and 868 men) found that higher levels of physical activity are associated with greater amounts of weight loss and a lower body weight. Individuals in the highest exercise group (burning more than 3,500 calories per week) weighed an average of 7.3 pounds less than those in the lowest physical activity group (burning less than 1,000 calories per week) and were maintaining a 9.2-pound greater weight loss at the time they entered the registry.

This emphasis on exercise among successful weight losers is not limited to the US. In a review of fifty-two research studies from the several weight control registries around the world (including US, Portugal, Germany, Finland, and Greece), increased physical activity was the most consistent factor that positively correlated to weight-loss maintenance.[170] Other research independent of the NWCR and international weight control registries has also shown the powerful effects of exercise in keeping weight off, and that high levels of physical activity are particularly important for being a successful weight loser.[171-178] One randomized clinical trial compared the effects of prescribing moderate or high levels of physical activity (1,000 calories per week vs. 2,500 calories per week) to 202 overweight individuals.[179] Weight loss was measured after six, twelve, and eighteen months. Not only did the 2,500-calorie-per-week group lose more weight after eighteen months compared to the 1,000-calorie-per-week group, the total amount of calories burned during exercise was strongly correlated with weight change.

One way to create the exercise habit is to exercise at the same time every day. One of the latest NWCR studies, published in *Obesity* in 2019, found that 68 percent of registry members were consistent in the timing of their exercise, with 47.8 percent being early-morning exercisers.[180] Exercising first thing in the morning may be especially conducive to fostering an exercise habit, since waking up may serve as a cue for initiating exercise. Although early morning is the most common time of day to exercise among successful weight losers, having greater consistency in habit-forming cues to exercise (e.g., exercising first thing upon getting out of bed or pairing leaving your workplace with going to the gym) and making exercise automatic are more important than the time of day. Whether NWCR members exercised early in the morning or in the evening was not related to the amount of exercise they did. Individuals who were consistent exercisers at the same time every day exercised more often, did longer workouts, and exercised at a higher intensity more often. They were also more likely to meet national exercise guidelines compared to individuals who were inconsistent in the timing of their exercise. As with the creation of most habits, you need to set the right environment to exercise.

When you exercise, you must be careful about not depositing the calories you just spent. Humans are excellent at balancing caloric expenses with caloric deposits. It's why overweight people have a hard time losing weight when they start exercising. As scientists at Montclair State University in New Jersey and the Pennington Biomedical Research Center in Baton Rouge, Louisiana, discovered after reviewing the exercise and weight-loss research, the small amount of weight loss observed from the majority of exercise intervention studies is primarily due to low doses of prescribed exercise, compounded by a concomitant increase in caloric intake.[181] In other words, people don't exercise enough, and they eat more to compensate for the calories they expend during exercise. People tend to eat more when they exercise more, especially aerobic exercise, like hiking, running, or cycling. Research as far back as 1956 published in *American Journal of Clinical Nutrition* has shown that people's caloric intake increases the more active they are.[182] But the converse is not true. Below a specific level of activity—what the scientists called the "sedentary zone"—a decrease in physical activity is not followed by a matched decrease in food intake but rather by an *increase*. People at the extreme ends of physical activity—those who exercise a lot and those who don't exercise at all—are the ones who eat the most.

I am often asked by people trying to lose weight how often they should exercise. While the best answer is that you only have to exercise on the days you eat, not everyone gets my sense of humor. But that answer is pretty close to the truth. If you aren't prepared to substantially increase your physical activity, your chances of being a successful weight loser are low. When you're physically active, you burn the fuel you consume, so it doesn't collect around your waist or on your thighs or, worse yet, around your abdominal organs as visceral fat. Trying to keep your weight off without increasing physical activity makes it practically impossible to relax your diet. When you exercise, your diet can be more flexible—you can eat a few chocolate chip cookies and it won't ruin your weight-loss or weight-maintenance goals; you can still become a successful weight loser. If you don't exercise, however, your diet becomes everything; no chocolate chip cookies allowed.

Successful weight loss requires more exercise to keep the weight off than what it takes to prevent excessive weight gain in the first place. People who don't exercise (or reduce how much exercise they do) are not only more likely to gain weight, it is inevitable that they will. A consistent, high level of exercise is one of the most important predictors of whether or not someone will be able to keep the weight off.[183] In one NWCR study on

3,591 of its members, while neither the amount of exercise, total daily calories consumed, nor percentage of calories from fat at the time they entered the registry predicted weight regain after three years, *changes* in these variables did predict weight regain.[184] Over the three years, 44 percent of individuals decreased the amount of exercise calories they burned by at least 500 calories per week, and 36 percent increased the amount of calories they consumed by at least 150 calories per day. Individuals who decreased exercise and increased calories consumed regained more weight. The combination of both had even greater consequences—those who decreased exercise *and* increased calories consumed regained the most weight over three years. The converse was also true: those who *increased* exercise and *decreased* calories consumed regained the least weight over three years.

To delve deeper into the characteristics and exercise habits of the NWCR, a study on 2,228 of its members divided them into clusters based on their characteristics and behaviors.[185] The researchers found that the NWCR members can be divided into four clusters. Cluster 1, which is made up of 50.5 percent, is the "Typical Members." They fit well with most of the characteristics of successful weight losers from the NWCR. They lost an average of 62.4 pounds and kept off the NWCR requirement of at least thirty pounds for an average of 5.8 years. They consume an average of 1,373 calories per day and do the most amount of exercise (2,853 calories per week). Their most common strategies for maintaining or losing weight include keeping many healthy foods in the house (96.6 percent of members), weighing on a regular basis (85.5 percent), and keeping few high-fat foods in the house (79.8 percent). More than a quarter (27.7 percent) say they can eat what they want and maintain weight. Cluster 2, which is made up of 26.9 percent, is the "Strugglers." They are more likely to have been obese as children, used more structured help to lose weight, and struggled the most to maintain their weight loss. Even so, they lost an average of 100.5 pounds, the most of all the clusters. They consume 1,457 calories per day and burn 2,492 calories per week during exercise. They were the least healthy of the four clusters before successful weight loss, with the highest prevalence of hypertension, high cholesterol, diabetes, sleep apnea, and major depression. Only 6.8 percent say they can eat what they want and maintain weight. Cluster 3, which is made up of 12.7 percent (and the highest percentage of men at 41.6 percent), are the "Stars." They are the polar opposite of Cluster 2. They have immediate and long-term success. Nearly all (94.8 percent) succeeded on their first try at weight loss. They lost an average of 56 pounds and kept off the NWCR requirement of at least thirty pounds for an average of 11.1 years, almost five years longer than any other cluster. They are the most weight-stable group, being the least likely to have been overweight as children or as adolescents, and the least likely to have an overweight family. They consume 1,419 calories per day and burn 2,661 calories per week. More than a third (36.8 percent) say they can eat what they want and maintain weight. Cluster 4, which is made up of 9.9 percent, is the "No Exercisers." They lost an average of 70.4 pounds but, although they are still successful weight losers, they don't engage in as many of the lifestyle behaviors as members of the other clusters, most notably exercise. They consume 1,352 calories per day and burn only 728 calories per week, far below that of other clusters, and don't use many other strategies to compensate, other than consuming fewer meals per day than members of the other clusters. When asked to rate the importance of following an exercise routine to maintain their weight on a scale of 1 (not important at all) to 8 (extremely important), the No Exercisers rate exercise at 3.2, while Clusters 1, 2, and 3 rate it much higher at 7.5, 7.4, and 7.3, respectively. Similar to the Stars of Cluster 3, 37.5 percent of No Exercisers say they can eat what they want and still maintain their weight.

While it may be easy or convenient to think that the reason why some people exercise and others don't is because the ones who do have the time and resources, like access to a gym or personal trainer, or because they simply like to exercise, the NWCR has shown that what makes a successful weight loser exercise has little to do with these factors. Whether or not someone exercises comes down to his or her commitment and the creation of and persistence in the habit. Remember habit 1? Live with intention. When you are serious and persistent in your commitment to keep the weight off and you have created the environmental cues to make the exercise habit unconscious, that intention will direct your behavior.

Creating the Habit

Contrary to creating dietary habits, creating exercise habits requires greater action. It's much easier to stop drinking soda or eat from a smaller plate than it is to run around the block or take a group fitness class at the gym. Perhaps the best way to create the habit of exercising (a lot) every day is to make the decision to be happier and live a more fulfilling life. That decision will direct your efforts. Strive toward a goal and to become a better version of yourself. Habit 1, Live with

Intention, is important here, so you must develop that habit first. Once you have created that habit, try these strategies:

1) Lay your workout clothes right next to your bed so you are encouraged to exercise first thing in the morning. Your workout clothes become a visual cue to exercise.

2) Exercise at the same time every day. Like for the majority of NWCR members who do so, exercising at the same time every day is a potent way to create a habit.

3) Find a friend to go to the gym with you, and make a regular, standing gym appointment with that friend.

4) Hire a personal trainer who can coach you through workouts and provide accountability, motivation, and inspiration.

5) Start small. You don't have to run a marathon the first week. Some exercise is better than no exercise, even just a ten-minute walk every other day. Remember, you are creating the habit. The more often you set time aside to do something physically active, even if it's for just a few minutes, you are training your brain to create the habit.

6) Set a timer at your office desk to ring every fifteen minutes. Every time you hear the ring, stand up from your chair and do twenty squats. Like Pavlov's dogs that salivated when hearing a bell because their brains were trained to think they were getting food, your brain will eventually associate "ring" with "squats," and you'll do it automatically. (Your coworkers may initially think you're a bit strange when they see you squatting to a timer, but soon you'll have them doing it, too!)

7) Cancel your cable TV service. Part of creating an exercise habit is becoming aware of and eliminating the habits that prevent you from exercising. Watching TV is one of the biggest exercise-preventing habits. There is a direct relationship between how much TV people watch and how little they exercise. If TV is no longer an option, that leaves you time to create the habit of exercise.

8) Always have a physical goal you're working toward. With a goal, exercise becomes training for the goal, rather than exercise for the sake of exercise. To steal a line from New York Yankees baseball player Yogi Berra, if you don't know where you're going, you might not get there. A goal provides you with the knowledge of where you're going.

9) Know your "why." The successful weight losers in the NWCR have reasons for being physically active that are connected to their personal values and mission and go far beyond reaching a number on a scale. Find a physical activity that you feel good doing, something that gives you confidence, something through which you feel self-acceptance.

**

"The experience of walking through that landscape—towering red canyon walls rising six hundred, eight hundred, one thousand feet, painted with streaks of black varnish deposited over thousands of years, deep sapphire sky above, and electric yellow cottonwood leaves—shifted something in me," Jamie Ash says. "The visual beauty of the place was astounding, but the experience of spending day after day moving, walking, breathing deeply was equally transformational." Jamie's previous experience with exercise was as something she felt she had to do to lose weight, a chore, something to get on the other side of as quickly as possible. But, hiking in Utah, Jamie discovered, was movement for the pleasure of it, which was altogether a different experience. "I fell in love with hiking, with being outside, and continued to hike after I got home," she says. When winter came a couple of months later, she got snowshoes so she could continue to hike.

After a few months of hiking, Jamie noticed that her clothes fit differently. When I started hiking as a way to move through a beautiful landscape, I had not thought of weight loss, let alone significant, lasting weight loss," she says. "Having been unsuccessful maintaining my previous weight loss, I thought it wasn't really possible for me and would likely end in disappointment and failure. Since I like to be successful, I chose not to try." Stepping on the scale for the first time in a year, she weighed less. "Not a lot less," she says, "maybe five pounds, but it was enough that I started to consider intentionally trying to lose weight."

Jamie changed the way she ate. She stopped going to her favorite place for enchiladas after she hiked. She stopped eating dessert. She learned portion control. She started counting calories. "I became aware of the difference between eating out of hunger and eating out of boredom, or proximity to the kitchen," she says. "I got comfortable with the sensation of hunger, not just eating because I liked to eat, and stopping before I was overly full." She also started counting hours per week hiking on the trail. The weight came off steadily, but, to her, it was a surprise. She weighed herself once per week. Every week, the number decreased by one, one and a half, sometimes two pounds.

As she lost weight, she read scientific articles for help and hints, and came across the NWCR. "I saw it was about maintaining weight, which was something I had never been able to do," she says. "I set a goal of becoming part of that database. My thinking was that by joining and receiving the annual surveys, I would be accountable to something outside of myself."

When Jamie's weight dropped to the mid-140s, she found herself in uncharted territory as an adult. "When I broke into the 130s, I didn't even know what to think," she says. "When I hit the 120s a year after starting to lose weight, well, I still get teary-eyed thinking about that. I never thought it was possible for my body to be as small or as strong as I was becoming. I could hike farther with less effort. I felt lithe, powerful, self-possessed. It felt like a treat every day to have the body I had."

In summer of 2019, Jamie's spouse was diagnosed with pancreatic cancer. They lived in nearby Albuquerque through December during radiation treatment. "I joined a gym during our time there, but I was doing about a third of the amount of exercise I'm used to," she says. To augment her spouse's weight loss from the cancer and treatment, Jamie cooked delicious, calorie-laden meals for both of them, including an evening meal of ice cream. "I went on an ice cream diet for that time," she says. "Much less weekly exercise and a high-fat, ice cream diet is not the way to maintain one's weight loss." After increasing to 132 pounds, the most she weighed in five years, she again noticed that her clothes were getting tight. She joined Weight Watchers since she felt she needed some structure to help her maintain the loss. She's now 128 pounds, working on getting back to 125 pounds. She has kept off 44 pounds for five years. It has taken a concerted effort, attention, and willingness to be hungry. "For the most part, the maintenance hasn't been that difficult, although I'm finding that shedding the six or so pounds I recently gained requires a strictness I'm not used to," she admits.

Exercise has been Jamie's biggest habit to maintain her weight. Lots of it. "My hiking has brought me access to experiences that seemed out of reach," she says. "It has also become a central strategy to reducing the stress of my spouse's pancreatic cancer." After a couple of years of hiking, she went on her first backpacking trip. She loved it so much that she started to go backpacking on her own. After her first solo backpacking trip, she signed up for a two-week backpacking and pack rafting trip to the Arrigetch Peaks. "If I had not maintained my weight loss, that trip would have been unthinkable," she says. Her odyssey even made it into *The Taos News*.

While training for a second trip to the Brooks Mountain Range in May 2019, Jamie fell and broke her ankle. "One of my first thoughts was how I could strategize to keep the weight off," she says. While on crutches, she got creative and exercised on the rowing machine at the gym with her broken leg crossed over her healthy leg. She also was careful to eat smaller portions and no sugar or desserts. With these strategies, she was able to maintain her weight loss through the injury.

Hiking has become central to Jamie's life and her identity, something that gives her much more than weight maintenance; it gives her solitude. "It's a different kind of solitude than simply having time alone in my house or time alone when I'm working," she says. "It's an expansive solitude."

When Jamie describes her hiking experience, she speaks with the eloquence of a philosopher. "Hiking alone gives me access to a kind of forest quiet: the gurgle of water running over rocks and fallen branches, the hammering of woodpeckers making themselves a roost in a tree, the wind blowing through pine boughs, sometimes soft and gentle, sometimes harsh and ferocious. It's full of physical challenge that I have come to love. As I hike in the Columbine-Hondo Wilderness, which climbs to over 12,000 feet of altitude, there's lots of walking uphill, which is never easy. It involves breathing hard, working my muscles, and the determination to get up high. Then there's a big payoff as I look down from a ridge or a summit to the mesas below or across the undulating ridges of mountains. It keeps me grounded, emotionally even, and walking for hours gives me lots of endorphins."

I finished my conversation with Jamie, now fifty-eight years old, by asking her what she wants others to know about maintaining weight loss and what advice she has to give. "Accept the fact that you are probably never going to be able to ignore calories and exercise," she says. "With sixty just a year and a half away, I'd like to think that all the exercise I do should allow me to eat whatever I want, but that is far from the reality.

"Make the experience of having a body that is easier to move and to live in be more important than the pleasure of eating. And find a physical activity you absolutely love and embrace it whole-heartedly. Let it become part of who you are, a self-expression."

HABIT 6

EXERCISE (A LOT) EVERY DAY.

Epilogue

The major conclusion of the NWCR is that successful weight losers adopt and persist with specific habits to totally restructure their eating and exercise behaviors. How they do it is not so much of a mystery. They live with intention and control themselves. The number of calories they eat, the amount of carbohydrate, fat, and protein they consume, how much they exercise, even how much television they watch, all extend from the first two habits of living with intention and controlling themselves.

When I started writing this book, I thought I was going to report the data from the NWCR that are hidden from public view in scientific journals, and let that be enough. "Here's what successful weight losers do," I was going to say, "now you figure out how to do it." But that's not enough. It's hard for data alone to inspire. They're just data.

The seven NWCR members featured in this book hope to personify the data and inspire you to make lasting change. Each of these people, and the thousands more who accompany them in the NWCR, have been able to convert the habits that made them overweight into habits that made them successful weight losers. That's not an easy thing to do.

To be a successful weight loser, you must reject all the popular media nonsense about weight loss and diets and accept that losing weight and keeping it off is hard work. Perhaps harder than anything else you have done in your life. That's okay. Life is hard. Just because it's hard doesn't mean you shouldn't do it or that you should give up after failing once or twice, or even after failing ten times. Anything in life worth pursuing is hard. If it were easy, it wouldn't be as fulfilling when you accomplish it. Despite the chance of failing, people take risks because the chance of failing makes success taste even sweeter. It is precisely in working through the difficulty that you reap the benefits that count the most.

There's more to becoming a successful weight loser than just becoming slimmer, although that alone would be enough for most people. When you dig deeper, there is something even more valuable than weighing less and looking better in the mirror. You learn about yourself. You learn what it means to do more, to be more, to do better, to be better.

When you set out to be a successful weight loser, clear of the doubts that hold you back, the payoff is extraordinary, no matter what the scale in your bathroom reads. But if you create and stick to the habits in this book, that scale will forever read lighter and, even more importantly, your life will change for the better. Just ask the successful weight losers of the National Weight Control Registry.

Acknowledgments

As I close the chapter on my tenth book, there are many people whom I'd like to thank...

Grace Freedson, my literary agent. Thank you for all the opportunities. It has been twelve years and ten books since I received your letter in my mailbox offering to represent me. Thank you for taking a chance.

Jack Karp, my twin brother and the best writer and editor I know, for inspiring me every day to view writing as art and for explaining to me, in the words of Hemingway, that "the first draft of anything is shit" and should be thrown out.

The editorial staff at Mango, for shaping this book into something that will help millions of people lose weight forever.

Dr. Rena Wing and Dr. James Hill, the founders of the National Weight Control Registry (NWCR), for the research you have done on this important topic. Without you, we would not have such a prolonged and thorough scientific evaluation of the habits of successful weight losers, and I wouldn't have had the idea to write this book.

Finally, thank you to the successful weight losers from the National Weight Control Registry, for showing the world that successful weight loss is indeed possible when you adopt and persist with the right habits. I am especially grateful for the NWCR members who were willing to share their inspiring stories that enrich this book and bring the data of the registry to life: Jamie Ash, Lynn Kata, Emily Kilar, Jeremy Kirkham, Diann Marten, Brenda Trosin, and Summer Yule. Thank you for sharing an important piece of your life. I hope your stories inspire others to do what you have done to become permanently lighter versions of themselves.

Endnotes

[1] Stunkard, A.J. and McLaren-Hume, M. The results of treatment for obesity: A review of the literature and report of a series. *Archives of Internal Medicine*, 103(1):79–85, 1959.

[2] American Society for Metabolic and Bariatric Surgery and National Opinion Research Center at the University of Chicago. New insights into Americans' perceptions and misperceptions of obesity treatments, and the struggles many face. *National Opinion Research Center at the University of Chicago (NORC)*, 1–13, 2016.

[3] Kramer, F.M., Jeffery, R.W., Forster, J.L., and Snell, M.K. Long-term follow-up of behavioral treatment for obesity: patterns of weight regain among men and women. *International Journal of Obesity*, 13:123–136, 1989.

[4] Wadden, T.A. Treatment of obesity by moderate and severe caloric restriction: results from clinical research trials. *Annals of Internal Medicine*, 119:688–693, 1993.

[5] Ouellette, J.A. and Wood, W. Habit and intention in everyday life: the multiple processes by which past behavior predicts future behavior. *Psychological Bulletin*, 124:54–74, 1998.

[6] American Society for Metabolic and Bariatric Surgery and National Opinion Research Center at the University of Chicago. New insights into Americans' perceptions and misperceptions of obesity treatments, and the struggles many face. *National*

Opinion Research Center at the University of Chicago (NORC), 1–13, 2016.

[7] Wood, W. *Good Habits, Bad Habits: The Science of Making Positive Changes that Stick.* New York: Farrar, Straus and Giroux, 2019.

[8] Olson, K.L., Lillis, J., Thomas, J.G., and Wing, R.R. Prospective evaluation of internalized weight bias and weight change among successful weight-loss maintainers. *Obesity*, 26(12):1888–1892, 2018.

[9] Christakis, N.A. and Fowler, J.H. The spread of obesity in a large social network over 32 years. *The New England Journal of Medicine*, 357:370–379, 2007.

[10] Hill, J.O., Wyatt, H.R., Phelan, S., and Wing, R.R. The National Weight Control Registry: Is it useful in helping deal with our obesity epidemic? *Journal of Nutrition Education and Behavior*, 37:206–210, 2005.

[11] Wing, R.R. and Hill, J.O. Successful weight loss maintenance. *Annual Review of Nutrition*, 21:323–341, 2001.

[12] Klem, M.L., Wing, R.R., McGuire, M.T., Seagle, H.M., and Hill, J.O. A descriptive study of individuals successful at long-term maintenance of substantial weight loss. *American Journal of Clinical Nutrition*, 66:239–246, 1997.

[13] McGuire, M.T., Wing, R.R., Klem, M.L., Seagle, H.M., and Hill, J.O. Long-term maintenance of weight loss: Do people who lose weight through various weight loss methods use

different behaviors to maintain their weight? *International Journal of Obesity*, 22:572–577, 1998.

[14] LaRose, J.G., Leahey, T.M., Hill, J.O., and Wing, R.R. Differences in motivations and weight loss behaviors in young adults and older adults in the National Weight Control Registry. *Obesity*, 21(3):449–453, 2013.

[15] McGuire, M.T., Wing, R.R., Klem, M.L., Lang, W., and Hill, J.O. What predicts weight regain among a group of successful weight losers? *Journal of Consulting and Clinical Psychology*, 67:177–185, 1999.

[16] Raynor, D., Phelan, S., Hill, J.O., and Wing, R.R. Television viewing and long-term weight maintenance: results from the National Weight Control Registry. *Obesity Research*, 14:1816–1824, 2006.

[17] Niemeier, H.M., Phelan, S., Fava, J.L., and Wing, R.R. Internal disinhibition predicts weight regain following weight loss and weight loss maintenance. *Obesity*, 15:2485–2494, 2007.

[18] Catenacci, V.A., Odgen, L., Phelan, S., Thomas, J.G., Hill, J.O., Wing, R.R., and Wyatt, H.R. Dietary habits and weight maintenance success in high versus low exercisers in the National Weight Control Registry. *Journal of Physical Activity and Health*, 11(8):1540–1548, 2014.

[19] Lillis, J., Thomas, J.G., Niemeier, H., and Wing, R.R. Internal disinhibition predicts 5-year weight regain in the National Weight Control Registry (NWCR). *Obesity Science & Practice*, 2(1):83–87, 2016.

[20] Thomas, J.G. and Wing, R.R. Maintenance of long-term weight loss. *Medicine and Health Rhode Island*, 92(2):56–57, 2009.

[21] McGuire, M.T., Wing, R.R., Klem, M.L., Lang, W., and Hill, J.O. What predicts weight regain among a group of successful weight losers? *Journal of Consulting and Clinical Psychology*, 67:177–185, 1999.

[22] Thomas, J.G., Bond, D.S., Phelan, S., Hill, J.O., and Wing, R.R. Weight-loss maintenance for 10 years in the National Weight Control Registry. *American Journal of Preventive Medicine*, 46(1):17–23, 2014.

[23] Gorin, A.A., Phelan, S., Hill, J.O., and Wing, R.R. Medical triggers are associated with better short- and long-term weight loss outcomes. *Preventive Medicine*, 39:612–616, 2004.

[24] McGuire, M.T., Wing, R.R., Klem, M.L., and Hill, J.O. Behavioral strategies of individuals who have maintained long-term weight losses. *Obesity Research*, 7:334–341, 1999.

[25] Wing, R.R. and Hill, J.O. Successful weight loss maintenance. *Annual Review of Nutrition*, 21:323–341, 2001.

[26] Phelan, S., Wing, R.R., Hill, J.O., and Dibello, J. Recovery from relapse among successful weight maintainers. *American Journal of Clinical Nutrition*, 78:1079–1084, 2003.

[27] McGuire, M.T., Wing, R.R., Klem, M.L., Lang, W., and Hill, J.O. What predicts weight regain among a group of successful weight losers? *Journal of Consulting and Clinical Psychology*, 67:177–185, 1999.

[28] Klem, M.L., Wing, R.R., Lang, W., McGuire, M.T., and Hill, J.O. Does weight loss maintenance become easier over time? *Obesity Research*, 8:438–444, 2000.

[29] McGuire, M.T., Wing, R.R., Klem, M.L., Lang, W., and Hill, J.O. What predicts weight regain among a group of successful weight losers? *Journal of Consulting and Clinical Psychology*, 67:177–185, 1999.

[30] Wing, R.R. and Hill, J.O. Successful weight loss maintenance. *Annual Review of Nutrition*, 21:323–341, 2001.

[31] Klem, M.L., Wing, R.R., Lang, W., McGuire, M.T., and Hill, J.O. Does weight loss maintenance become easier over time? *Obesity Research*, 8:438–444, 2000.

[32] Gold, J.M., Carr, L.J., Thomas, J.G., Burrus, J., O'Leary, K.C., Wing, R., and Bond, D.S. Conscientiousness in weight loss maintainers and regainers. *Health Psychology*, 39(5):421-429, 2020.

[33] Ajzen, I. The theory of planned behavior. *Organizational Behavior and Human Decision Processes*, 50(2):179–211, 1991.

[34] Bandura, A. *Social Foundations of Thought and Action: A Social Cognitive Theory*. Englewood Cliffs, NJ: Prentice-Hall, 1986.

[35] Godin, G. and Kok, G. The theory of planned behavior: a review of its applications to health-related behaviors. *American Journal of Health Promotion*, 11(2):87–98, 1996.

[36] Vroom, V.H. *Work and Motivation*. New York: Wiley, 1964.

37 Kuijer, R.G. and Boyce, J.A. Chocolate cake. Guilt or celebration? Associations with healthy eating attitudes, perceived behavioral control, intentions and weight-loss. *Appetite*, 74:48–54, 2014.

38 Mischel, W., Ebbesen, E.B., and Zeiss, A.R. Cognitive and attentional mechanisms in delay of gratification. *Journal of Personality and Social Psychology*, 21(2):204–218, 1972.

39 Mischel, W. and Ebbesen, E.B. Attention in delay of gratification. *Journal of Personality and Social Psychology*, 16(2):329–337, 1970.

40 McGuire, M.T., Wing, R.R., Klem, M.L., Lang, W. and Hill, J.O. What predicts weight regain among a group of successful weight losers? *Journal of Consulting and Clinical Psychology*, 67:177–185, 1999.

41 Niemeier, H.M., Phelan, S., Fava, J.L., and Wing, R.R. Internal disinhibition predicts weight regain following weight loss and weight loss maintenance. *Obesity*, 15:2485–2494, 2007.

42 Butryn, M.L., Phelan, S., Hill, J.O., and Wing, R.R. Consistent self-monitoring of weight: A key component of successful weight loss maintenance. *Obesity*, 15:3091–3096, 2007.

43 Thomas, J.G., Bond, D.S., Phelan, S., Hill, J.O., and Wing, R.R. Weight-loss maintenance for 10 years in the National Weight Control Registry. *American Journal of Preventive Medicine*, 46(1):17–23, 2014.

44 Lillis, J., Thomas, J.G., Niemeier, H., and Wing, R.R. Internal disinhibition predicts 5-year weight regain in the

National Weight Control Registry (NWCR). *Obesity Science and Practice*, 2(1):83–87, 2016.

45 Poulimeneas, D., Yannakoulia, M., Anastasiou, C.A., and Scarmeas, N. Weight loss maintenance: Have we missed the brain? *Brain Sciences*, 8(174):1–10, 2018.

46 Niemeier, H.M., Phelan, S., Fava, J.L., and Wing, R.R. Internal disinhibition predicts weight regain following weight loss and weight loss maintenance. *Obesity*, 15:2485–2494, 2007.

47 Lillis, J., Thomas, J.G., Niemeier, H., and Wing, R.R. Internal disinhibition predicts 5-year weight regain in the National Weight Control Registry (NWCR). *Obesity Science and Practice*, 2(1):83–87, 2016.

48 Drapkin, R.G., Wing, R.R., and Shiffman, S. Responses to hypothetical high risk situations: do they predict weight loss in a behavioral treatment program or the context of dietary lapses? *Health Psychology*, 14:427–434, 1995.

49 Grilo, C.M., Shiffman, S., and Wing, R.R. Relapse crises and coping among dieters. *Journal of Consulting and Clinical Psychology*, 57:488–495, 1989.

50 Carels, R.A., Hoffman, J., Collins, A., Raber, A.C., Cacciapaglia, H., and O'Brien, W.H. Ecological momentary assessment of temptation and lapse in dieting. *Eating Behaviors*, 2:307–321, 2001.

51 Carels, R.A., Douglass, O.M., Cacciapaglia, H.M., and O'Brien, W.H. An ecological momentary assessment of relapse crises

in dieting. *Journal of Consulting and Clinical Psychology*, 72:341–348, 2004.

[52] Byrne, S., Cooper, Z., and Fairburn, C. Weight maintenance and relapse in obesity: a qualitative study. *International Journal of Obesity and Related Metabolic Disorders*, 27:955–962, 2003.

[53] Bickel, W.K., Moody, L.N., Koffarnus, M., Thomas, J.G., and Wing, R. Self-control as measured by delay discounting is greater among successful weight losers than controls. *Journal of Behavioral Medicine*, 41(6):891–896, 2018.

[54] Chamberlain, S.R., Derbyshire, K.L., Leppink, E., and Grant, J.E. Obesity and dissociable forms of impulsivity in young adults. *CNS Spectrums*, 20(5):500–507, 2015.

[55] Fields, S.A., Sabet, M., and Reynolds, B. Dimensions of impulsive behavior in obese, overweight, and healthy-weight adolescents. *Appetite*, 70:60–66, 2013.

[56] Amlung, M., Petker, T., Jackson, J., Balodis, I., and MacKillop, J. Steep discounting of delayed monetary and food rewards in obesity: a meta-analysis. *Psychological Medicine*, 46(11):2423–2434, 2016.

[57] Kanfer, F.H. and Karoly, P. Self-control: a behavioristic excursion into the lion's den. *Behavior Therapy*, 3:398–416, 1972.

[58] Kirschenbaum, D.S. Self-regulatory failure: a review with clinical implications. *Clinical Psychology Review*, 7:77–104, 1987.

[59] Wing, R.R. and Phelan, S. Long-term weight loss maintenance. *American Journal of Clinical Nutrition*, 82:222S–225S, 2005.

[60] Wing, R.R. and Hill, J.O. Successful weight loss maintenance. *Annual Review of Nutrition*, 21:323–341, 2001.

[61] Wyatt, H.R., Phelan, S., Wing, R.R., and Hill, J.O. Lessons from patients who have successfully maintained weight loss. *Obesity Management*, 1:56–61, 2005.

[62] Butryn, M.L., Phelan, S., Hill, J.O., and Wing, R.R. Consistent self-monitoring of weight: a key component of successful weight loss maintenance. *Obesity*, 15:3091–3096, 2007.

[63] Bickel, W.K., Moody, L.N., Koffarnus, M., Thomas, J.G., and Wing, R. Self-control as measured by delay discounting is greater among successful weight losers than controls. *Journal of Behavioral Medicine*, 41(6):891–896, 2018.

[64] Wing, R.R. and Phelan, S. Long-term weight loss maintenance. *American Journal of Clinical Nutrition*, 82:222S–225S, 2005.

[65] Wing, R.R. and Hill, J.O. Successful weight loss maintenance. *Annual Review of Nutrition*, 21:323–341, 2001.

[66] Butryn, M.L., Phelan, S., Hill, J.O., and Wing, R.R. Consistent self-monitoring of weight: A key component of successful weight loss maintenance. *Obesity*, 15:3091–3096, 2007.

67 McGuire, M.T., Wing, R.R., Klem, M.L., and Hill, J.O. Behavioral strategies of individuals who have maintained long-term weight losses. *Obesity Research*, 7:334–341, 1999.

68 Goldstein, C.M., Thomas, J.G., Wing, R.R., and Bond, D.S. Successful weight loss maintainers use health-tracking smartphone applications more than a nationally representative sample: comparison of the National Weight Control Registry to Pew Tracking for Health. *Obesity Science and Practice*, 3(2):117–126, 2017.

69 Neal, D.T., Wood, W., Wu, M., and Kurlander, D. The pull of the past: When do habits persist despite conflict with motives? *Personality and Social Psychology Bulletin*, 37(11):1428–1437, 2011.

70 Mahoney, M.J. and Avener, M. Psychology of the elite athlete: An exploratory study. *Cognitive Therapy and Research*, 1:135–141, 1977.

71 Meyers, A.W., Cooke, C.J., Cullen, J., and Liles, L. Psychological aspects of athletic competitors: A replication across sports. *Cognitive Therapy and Research*, 3:361–366, 1979.

72 Kirschenbaum, D.S. and Bale, R.M. Cognitive-behavioral skills in golf: Brain power golf. In R.M. Suinn (Ed.). *Psychology in Sports: Methods and Applications*. Minneapolis, MN: Burgess.

73 Gould, D., Weiss, M., and Weinberg, R. Psychological characteristics of successful and nonsuccessful Big Ten wrestlers. *Journal of Sport and Exercise Psychology*, 3(1):69–81, 1981.

74 Highlen, P.S. and Bennett, B.B. Elite divers and wrestlers: A comparison between open- and closed-skill athletes. *Journal of Sport and Exercise Psychology*, 5(4):390–409, 1983.

75 Sobal, J. and Wansink, B. Kitchenscapes, tablescapes, platescapes, and foodscapes: Influences of microscale built environments on food intake. *Environment and Behavior*, 39:124–142, 2007.

76 Wansink, B. and Kim, J. Bad popcorn in big buckets: portion size can influence intake as much as taste. *Journal of Nutrition Education and Behavior*, 37(5):242–245, 2005.

77 Marchiori, D., Corneille, O., and Klein, O. Container size influences snack food intake independently of portion size. *Appetite*, 58(3):814–817, 2012.

78 Klem, M.L., Wing, R.R., McGuire, M.T., Seagle, H.M., and Hill, J.O. A descriptive study of individuals successful at long-term maintenance of substantial weight loss. *American Journal of Clinical Nutrition*, 66:239–246, 1997.

79 Wing, R.R. and Hill, J.O. Successful weight loss maintenance. *Annual Review of Nutrition*, 21:323–341, 2001.

80 Shick, S.M., Wing, R.R., Klem, M.L., McGuire, M.T., Hill, J.O., and Seagle, H.M. Persons successful at long-term weight loss and maintenance continue to consume a low-energy, low-fat diet. *Journal of the American Dietetic Association*, 98:408–413, 1998.

81 McGuire, M.T., Wing, R.R., Klem, M.L., Seagle, H.M., and Hill, J.O. Long-term maintenance of weight loss: Do people

who lose weight through various weight loss methods use different behaviors to maintain their weight? *International Journal of Obesity*, 22:572–577, 1998.

[82] Klem, M.L., Wing, R.R., Chang, C.H., Lang, W., McGuire, M.T., Sugerman, H.J., Hutchison, S.L., Makovich, A.L., and Hill, J.O. A case-control study of successful maintenance of a substantial weight loss: Individuals who lost weight through surgery versus those who lost weight through nonsurgical means. *International Journal of Obesity*, 24:573–579, 2000.

[83] Klem, M.L., Wing, R.R., Lang, W., McGuire, M.T., and Hill, J.O. Does weight loss maintenance become easier over time? *Obesity Research*, 8:438–444, 2000.

[84] Ogden, L.G., Stroebele, N., Wyatt, H.R., Catenacci, V.A., Peters, J.C., Stuht, J., Wing, R.R., and Hill, J.O. Cluster analysis of the National Weight Control Registry to identify distinct subgroups maintaining successful weight loss. *Obesity*, 20(10):2039–2047, 2012.

[85] Wing, R.R. and Phelan, S. Long-term weight loss maintenance. *American Journal of Clinical Nutrition*, 82:222S–225S, 2005.

[86] Wright J.D., Wang, C.Y., Kennedy-Stephenson, J., and Ervin, R.B. Dietary intake of ten key nutrients for public health, United States: 1999–2000. *Advance Data From Vital and Health Statistics*, 334:1–4, 2003.

[87] U.S. Department of Agriculture, Agricultural Research Service. Energy intakes: percentages of energy from protein, carbohydrate, fat, and alcohol, by gender and age. *What We Eat in America, NHANES 2015–2016*, 2018.

[88] Katahn, M., Pleas, J., Thackery, M., and Wallston, K.A. Relationship of eating and activity self-reports to follow-up weight maintenance in the massively obese. *Behavior Therapy*, 13:521–528, 1982.

[89] Santos, I., Vieira, P.N., Silva, M.N., Sardinha, L.B., and Teixeira, P.J. Weight control behaviors of highly successful weight loss maintainers: the Portuguese Weight Control Registry. *Journal of Behavioral Medicine*, 40(2):366–371, 2017.

[90] Cornaro, L. *Discorsi Della Vita Sobria (Discourses on the Sober Life)*. New York: Crowell, 2007.

[91] McDonald, R.B. and Ramsey, J.J. Honoring Clive McCay and 75 years of calorie restriction research. *Journal of Nutrition*, 140(7):1205–1210, 2010.

[92] Wolfson, J.A. and Bleich, S.N. Is cooking at home associated with better diet quality or weight-loss intention? *Public Health Nutrition*, 18(8):1397–406, 2015.

[93] Wing, R.R. and Hill, J.O. Successful weight loss maintenance. *Annual Review of Nutrition*, 21:323–341, 2001.

[94] Thomas, J.G. and Wing, R.R. Maintenance of long-term weight loss. *Medicine & Health Rhode Island*, 92(2):56–57, 2009.

[95] Catenacci, V.A., Pan, Z., Thomas, J.G., Ogden, L.G., Roberts, S.A., Wyatt, H.R., Wing, R.R., and Hill, J.O. Low/no calorie sweetened beverage consumption in the National Weight Control Registry. *Obesity*, 22(10):2244–2251, 2014.

[96] Leibel, R.L. and Hirsch, J. Diminished energy requirements in reduced-obese patients. *Metabolism*, 33(2):164–170, 1984.

[97] Larson, D.E., Ferraro, R.T., Robertson, D.S., and Ravussin, E. Energy metabolism in weight-stable postobese individuals. *American Journal of Clinical Nutrition*, 62:735–739, 1995.

[98] Lean, M.E.J. and James, W.P.T. Metabolic effects of isoenergetic nutrient exchange over 24 hours in relation to obesity in women. *International Journal of Obesity*, 12:15–27, 1987.

[99] Leibel, R.L., Rosenbaum, M., and Hirsch, J. Changes in energy expenditure resulting from altered body weight. *New England Journal of Medicine*, 332(10):621–628, 1995.

[100] Camps, S.G.J.A., Verhoef, S.P.M., and Westerterp, K.R. Weight loss, weight maintenance, and adaptive thermogenesis. *American Journal of Clinical Nutrition*, 97:990–994, 2013.

[101] Astrup, A., Gotzsche, P.C., van de Werken, K., Ranneries, C., Toubro, S., Raben, A., and Buemann, B. Meta-analysis of resting metabolic rate in formerly obese subjects. *American Journal of Clinical Nutrition*, 69:1117–1122, 1999.

[102] Fothergill, E., Guo, J., Howard, L., Kerns, J.C., Knuth, N.D., Brychta, R., Chen, K.Y., Skarulis, M.C., Walter, M., Walter, P.J., and Hall, K.D. Persistent metabolic adaptation 6 years after "The Biggest Loser" competition. *Obesity*, 24:1612–1619, 2016.

[103] Wyatt, H.R., Grunwald, G.K., Seagle, H.M., Klem, M.L., McGuire, M.T., Wing, R.R., and Hill, J.O. Resting energy expenditure in reduced-obese subjects in the National Weight

Control Registry. *American Journal of Clinical Nutrition*, 69:1189–1193, 1999.

104 Raben, A., Andersen, H.B., Christensen, N.J., Madsen, J., Holst, J.J., and Astrup, A. Evidence for an abnormal postprandial response to a high-fat meal in women predisposed to obesity. *American Journal of Physiology*, 267:E549-E559, 1994.

105 Astrup, A. Dietary composition, substrate balances and body fat in subjects with a predisposition to obesity. *International Journal of Obesity and Related Metabolic Disorders*, 17:S32-S36, 1993.

106 Astrup, A., Buemann, B., Christensen, N.J., and Toubro, S. Failure to increase lipid oxidation in response to increasing dietary fat content in formerly obese women. *American Journal of Physiology*, 266:E592-E599, 1994.

107 Phelan, S., Wing, R.R., Raynor, H.A., Dibello, J., Nedeau, K., and Peng, W. Holiday weight management by successful weight losers and normal weight individuals. *Journal of Consulting and Clinical Psychology*, 76(3):442–448, 2008.

108 Shick, S.M., Wing, R.R., Klem, M.L., McGuire, M.T., Hill, J.O., and Seagle, H.M. Persons successful at long-term weight loss and maintenance continue to consume a low-energy, low-fat diet. *Journal of the American Dietetic Association*, 98:408–413, 1998.

109 McGuire, M.T., Wing, R.R., Klem, M.L., Seagle, H.M., and Hill, J.O. Long-term maintenance of weight loss: Do people who lose weight through various weight loss methods use

different behaviors to maintain their weight? *International Journal of Obesity*, 22:572–577, 1998.

[110] Klem, M.L., Wing, R.R., Chang, C.H., Lang, W., McGuire, M.T., Sugerman, H.J., Hutchison, S.L., Makovich, A.L., and Hill, J.O. A case-control study of successful maintenance of a substantial weight loss: Individuals who lost weight through surgery versus those who lost weight through nonsurgical means. *International Journal of Obesity*, 24:573–579, 2000.

[111] Klem, M.L., Wing, R.R., Lang, W., McGuire, M.T., and Hill, J.O. Does weight loss maintenance become easier over time? *Obesity Research*, 8:438–444, 2000.

[112] Wing, R.R. and Hill, J.O. Successful weight loss maintenance. *Annual Review of Nutrition*, 21:323–341, 2001.

[113] Phelan, S., Wyatt, H.R., Hill, J.O., and Wing, R.R. Are the eating and exercise habits of successful weight losers changing? *Obesity Research*, 14:710–716, 2006.

[114] LaRose, J.G., Leahey, T.M., Hill, J.O., and Wing, R.R. Differences in motivations and weight loss behaviors in young adults and older adults in the National Weight Control Registry. *Obesity*, 21(3):449–453, 2013.

[115] Bond, D.S., Phelan, S., Leahey, T.M., Hill, J.O., and Wing, R.R. Weight-loss maintenance in successful weight losers: surgical vs nonsurgical methods. *International Journal of Obesity*, 33:173–180, 2009.

[116] Harris, J.K., French, S.A., Jeffery, R.W., McGovern, P.G. and Wing, R.R. Dietary and physical activity correlates of long-term weight loss. *Obesity Research*, 2:307–313, 1994.

[117] Wing, R.R., Sinha, M., Considine, R., Lang, W., and Caro, J. Relationship between weight loss maintenance and changes in serum leptin levels. *Hormone and Metabolic Research*, 28:698–703, 1996.

[118] McGuire, M.T., Wing, R.R., Klem, M.L., and Hill, J.O. Behavioral strategies of individuals who have maintained long-term weight losses. *Obesity Research*, 7:334–341, 1999.

[119] French, S.A., Jeffery, R.W., Forster, J.L., McGovern, P.G., Kelder, S.H., and Baxter, J. Predictors of weight change over two years among a population of working adults: The Healthy Worker Project. *International Journal of Obesity and Related Metabolic Disorders*, 18(3):145–154, 1994.

[120] Phelan, S., Wyatt, H.R., Hill, J.O., and Wing, R.R. Are the eating and exercise habits of successful weight losers changing? *Obesity Research*, 14:710–716, 2006.

[121] Raynor, D., Phelan, S., Hill, J.O., and Wing, R.R. Television viewing and long-term weight maintenance: results from the National Weight Control Registry. *Obesity Research*, 14:1816–1824, 2006.

[122] Wing, R.R. and Hill, J.O. Successful weight loss maintenance. *Annual Review of Nutrition*, 21:323–341, 2001.

[123] Coyle, E.F. Carbohydrate supplementation during exercise. *Journal of Nutrition*, 122(Suppl. 3):788–795, 1992.

[124] Phelan, S., Wyatt, H.R., DiBello, J., Fava, J.L., Hill, J.O., and Wing, R.R. Three-year weight change in successful weight losers who lost weight on a low-carbohydrate diet. *Obesity,* 15:2470–2477, 2007.

[125] Foster, G.D., Wyatt, H.R., Hill, J.O., McGuckin, B.G., Brill, C., Mohammed, B.S., Szapary, P.O., Rader, D.J., Edman, J.S., and Klein, S. A randomized trial of a low-carbohydrate diet for obesity. *The New England Journal of Medicine,* 348(21):2082–2090, 2003.

[126] Soenen, S., Bonomi, A.G., Lemmens, S.G., Scholte, J., Thijssen, M.A., van Berkum, F., and Westerterp-Plantenga, M.S. Relatively high-protein or 'low-carb' energy-restricted diets for body weight loss and body weight maintenance? *Physiology & Behavior,* 107(3):374–380, 2012.

[127] McGuire, M.T., Wing, R.R., Klem, M.L., Lang, W., and Hill, J.O. What predicts weight regain among a group of successful weight losers? *Journal of Consulting and Clinical Psychology,* 67:177–185, 1999.

[128] An, R. and Burd, N.A. Change in daily energy intake associated with pairwise compositional change in carbohydate, fat and protein intake among US adults, 1999–2010. *Public Health Nutrition,* 18(8):1343–1352, 2015.

[129] Gorin, A.A., Phelan, S., Wing, R.R., and Hill, J.O. Promoting long-term weight control: does dieting consistency matter? *International Journal of Obesity and Related Metabolic Disorders,* 28:278–281, 2004.

[130] Raynor, H., Wing, R.R., and Phelan, S. Amount of food group variety consumed in the diet and long-term weight loss maintenance. *Obesity Research*, 13:883–890, 2005.

[131] Wyatt, H.R., Grunwald, O.K., Mosca, C.L., Klem, M.L., Wing, R.R., and Hill, J.O. Long-term weight loss and breakfast in subjects in the National Weight Control Registry. *Obesity Research*, 10:78–82, 2002.

[132] Santos, I., Vieira, P.N., Silva, M.N., Sardinha, L.B., and Teixeira, P.J. Weight control behaviors of highly successful weight loss maintainers: the Portuguese Weight Control Registry. *Journal of Behavioral Medicine*, 40(2):366–371, 2017.

[133] Haines, P.S., Guilkey, D.K., and Popkin, B.M. Trends in breakfast consumption of US adults between 1965 and 1991. *Journal of the American Dietetic Association*, 96(5):464–470, 1996.

[134] Farshchi, H.R., Taylor, M.A., and Macdonald, I.A. Deleterious effects of omitting breakfast on insulin sensitivity and fasting lipid profiles in healthy lean women. *American Journal of Clinical Nutrition*, 81(2):388–396, 2005.

[135] Cho, S., Dietrich, M., Brown, C.J., Clark, C.A., and Block, G. The effect of breakfast type on total daily energy intake and body mass index: results from the Third National Health and Nutrition Examination Survey (NHANES III). *Journal of the American College of Nutrition*, 22(4):296–302, 2003.

[136] Garaulet, M., Gómez-Abellán, P., Alburquerque-Béjar, J.J., Lee, Y.C., Ordovás, J.M., and Scheer, F.A. Timing of food intake

predicts weight loss effectiveness. *International Journal of Obesity*, 37(4):604–611, 2013.

[137] Jakubowicz, D., Barnea, M., Wainstein, J., and Froy, O. High caloric intake at breakfast vs. dinner differentially influences weight loss of overweight and obese women. *Obesity*, 21(12):2504–2512, 2013.

[138] Jakubowicz, D., Froy, O., Wainstein, J., and Boaz, M. Meal timing and composition influence ghrelin levels, appetite scores, and weight loss maintenance in overweight and obese adults. *Steroids*, 77(4):323–331, 2012.

[139] Ladabaum, U., Mannalithara, A., Myer, P.A., and Singh, G. Obesity, abdominal obesity, physical activity, and caloric intake in US adults: 1988 to 2010. *The American Journal of Medicine*, 127(8):717–727, 2014.

[140] Raynor, D., Phelan, S., Hill, J.O., and Wing, R.R. Television viewing and long-term weight maintenance: results from the National Weight Control Registry. *Obesity Research*, 14:1816–1824, 2006.

[141] Nielson Media Research. *Nielson Report on Television*. New York, NY: Nielson Media Research, 2000.

[142] Catenacci, V.A., Odgen, L., Phelan, S., Thomas, J.G., Hill, J.O., Wing, R.R., and Wyatt, H.R. Dietary habits and weight maintenance success in high versus low exercisers in the National Weight Control Registry. *Journal of Physical Activity and Health*, 11(8):1540–1548, 2014.

[143] Klem, M.L., Wing, R.R., McGuire, M.T., Seagle, H.M., and Hill, J.O. Psychological symptoms in individuals successful at long-term maintenance of weight loss. *Health Psychology*, 17:336–345, 1998.

[144] McGuire, M.T., Wing, R.R., Klem, M.L., Seagle, H.M., and Hill, J.O. Long-term maintenance of weight loss: Do people who lose weight through various weight loss methods use different behaviors to maintain their weight? *International Journal of Obesity*, 22:572–577, 1998.

[145] Klem, M.L., Wing, R.R., McGuire, M.T., Seagle, H.M., and Hill, J.O. Psychological symptoms in individuals successful at long-term maintenance of weight loss. *Health Psychology*, 17:336–345, 1998.

[146] Klem, M.L., Wing, R.R., Chang, C.H., Lang, W., McGuire, M.T., Sugerman, H.J., Hutchison, S.L., Makovich, A.L., and Hill, J.O. A case-control study of successful maintenance of a substantial weight loss: Individuals who lost weight through surgery versus those who lost weight through nonsurgical means. *International Journal of Obesity*, 24:573–579, 2000.

[147] Wing, R.R. and Hill, J.O. Successful weight loss maintenance. *Annual Review of Nutrition*, 21:323–341, 2001.

[148] Wyatt, H.R., Phelan, S., Wing, R.R., and Hill, J.O. Lessons from patients who have successfully maintained weight loss. *Obesity Management*, 1:56–61, 2005.

[149] Phelan, S., Wyatt, H.R., DiBello, J., Fava, J.L., Hill, J.O., and Wing, R.R. Three-year weight change in successful weight

losers who lost weight in a low-carbohydrate diet. *Obesity*, 15:2470–2477, 2007.

[150] Catenacci, V.A., Ogden, L.G., Stuht, J., Phelan, S., Wing, R.R., Hill, J.O., and Wyatt, H.R. Physical Activity patterns in the National Weight Control Registry. *Obesity*, 16:153–161, 2008.

[151] Ogden, L.G., Stroebele, N., Wyatt, H.R., Catenacci, V.A., Peters, J.C., Stuht, J., Wing, R.R., and Hill, J.O. Cluster analysis of the National Weight Control Registry to identify distinct subgroups maintaining successful weight loss. *Obesity*, 20(10):2039–2047, 2012.

[152] Donnelly, J.E., Blair, S.N., Jakicic, J.M., Manore, M.M., Rankin, J.W., and Smith, B.K. American College of Sports Medicine Position Stand. Appropriate physical activity intervention strategies for weight loss and prevention of weight regain for adults. *Medicine and Science in Sports and Exercise*, 41(2):459–471, 2009.

[153] Wing, R.R. and Hill, J.O. Successful weight loss maintenance. *Annual Review of Nutrition*, 21:323–341, 2001.

[154] Catenacci, V.A., Odgen, L., Phelan, S., Thomas, J.G., Hill, J.O., Wing, R.R., and Wyatt, H.R. Dietary habits and weight maintenance success in high versus low exercisers in the National Weight Control Registry. *Journal of Physical Activity and Health*, 11(8):1540–1548, 2014.

[155] Catenacci, V.A., Ogden, L.G., Stuht, J., Phelan, S., Wing, R.R., Hill, J.O., and Wyatt, H.R. Physical activity patterns in the National Weight Control Registry. *Obesity*, 16:153–161, 2008.

156 Catenacci, V.A., Grunwald, G.K., Ingebrigtsen, J.P., Jakicic, J.M., McDermott, M.D., Phelan, S., Wing, R.R., Hill, J.O., and Wyatt, H.R. Physical activity patterns using accelerometry in the National Weight Control Registry. *Obesity*, 19(6):1163–1170, 2011.

157 Phelan, S., Roberts, M., Lang, W., and Wing, R.R. Empirical evaluation of physical activity recommendations for weight control in women. *Medicine & Science in Sports & Exercise*, 39:1832–1836, 2007.

158 Thomas, J.G. and Wing, R.R. Maintenance of long-term weight loss. *Medicine & Health Rhode Island*, 92(2):56–57, 2009.

159 Wyatt, H.R., Phelan, S., Wing, R.R., and Hill, J.O. Lessons from patients who have successfully maintained weight loss. *Obesity Management*, 1:56–61, 2005.

160 Catenacci, V.A., Ogden, L.G., Stuht, J., Phelan, S., Wing, R.R., Hill, J.O., and Wyatt, H.R. Physical activity patterns in the National Weight Control Registry. *Obesity*, 16:153–161, 2008.

161 Wing, R.R. and Hill, J.O. Successful weight loss maintenance. *Annual Review of Nutrition*, 21:323–341, 2001.

162 Ibid.

163 Klem, M.L., Wing, R.R., Chang, C.H., Lang, W., McGuire, M.T., Sugerman, H.J., Hutchison, S.L., Makovich, A.L., and Hill, J.O. A case-control study of successful maintenance of a substantial weight loss: Individuals who lost weight through

surgery versus those who lost weight through nonsurgical means. *International Journal of Obesity*, 24:573–579, 2000.

[164] Ibid.

[165] Wardle, J., Carnell, S., Haworth, C.M., and Plomin, R. Evidence for a strong genetic influence on childhood adiposity despite the force of the obesogenic environment. *American Journal of Clinical Nutrition*, 87(2):398–404, 2008.

[166] Musani, S.K., Erickson, S., and Allison, D.B. Obesity—still highly heritable after all these years. *American Journal of Clinical Nutrition*, 87:275–276, 2008.

[167] McGuire, M.T., Wing, R.R., Klem, M.L., Lang, W., and Hill, J.O. What predicts weight regain among a group of successful weight losers? *Journal of Consulting and Clinical Psychology*, 67:177–185, 1999.

[168] Wing, R.R. and Hill, J.O. Successful weight loss maintenance. *Annual Review of Nutrition*, 21:323–341, 2001.

[169] Catenacci, V.A., Ogden, L.G., Stuht, J., Phelan, S., Wing, R.R., Hill, J.O., and Wyatt, H.R. Physical activity patterns in the National Weight Control Registry. *Obesity*, 16:153–161, 2008.

[170] Paixão, C., Dias, C.M., Jorge, R., Carraça, E.V., Yannakoulia, M., de Zwaan, M., Soini, S., Hill, J.O., Teixeira, P.J., and Santos, I. Successful weight loss maintenance: A systematic review of weight control registries. *Obesity Reviews*, 21(5):e13003, 2020.

44444

[171] Williams, P.T. and Thompson, P.D. Dose-dependent effects of training and detraining on weight in 6406 runners during 7.4 years. *Obesity*, 14:1975–1984, 2006.

[172] Curioni, C.C. and Lourenço, P.M. Long-term weight loss after diet and exercise: a systematic review. *International Journal of Obesity*, 29(10):1168–1174, 2005.

[173] Zachwieja, J.J. Exercise as treatment for obesity. *Endocrinology and Metabolism Clinics of North America*, 25(4):965–988, 1996.

[174] Wang, X., Lyles, M.F., You, T., Berry, M.J., Rejeski, W.J., and Nicklas, B.J. Weight regain is related to decreases in physical activity during weight loss. *Medicine & Science in Sports & Exercise*, 40(10):1781–1788, 2008.

[175] Crawford, D., Jeffery, R.W., and French, S.A. Can anyone successfully control their weight? Findings of a three year community-based study of men and women. *International Journal of Obesity and Related Metabolic Disorders*, 24(9):1107–1110, 2000.

[176] Kayman, S., Bruvold, W., and Stern, J.S. Maintenance and relapse after weight loss in women: behavioral aspects. *American Journal of Clinical Nutrition*, 52:800–807, 1990.

[177] Schoeller, D.A., Shay, K., and Kushner, R.F. How much physical activity is needed to minimize weight gain in previously obese women? *American Journal of Clinical Nutrition*, 66:551–556, 1997.

[178] Fogelholm, M., Kukkonen-Harjula, K., and Oja, P. Eating control and physical activity as determinants of short-term weight maintenance after a very-low-calorie diet among obese women. *International Journal of Obesity and Related Metabolic Disorders*, 23(2):203–210, 1999.

[179] Jeffery, R.W., Wing, R.R., Sherwood, N.E., and Tate, D.F. Physical activity and weight loss: does prescribing higher physical activity goals improve outcome? *American Journal of Clinical Nutrition*, 78:684–689, 2003.

[180] Schumacher, L.M., Thomas, J.G., Raynor, H.A., Rhodes, R.E., O'Leary, K.C., Wing, R.R., and Bond, D.S. Relationship of consistency in timing of exercise performance and exercise levels among successful weight loss maintainers. *Obesity*, 27(8):1285–1291, 2019.

[181] Thomas, D.M., Bouchard, C., Church, T., Slentz, C., Kraus, W.E., Redman, L.M., Martin, C.K., Silva, A.M., Vossen, M., Westerterp, K., and Heymsfield, S.B. Why do individuals not lose more weight from an exercise intervention at a defined dose? An energy balance analysis. *Obesity Reviews*, 13(10):835–847, 2012.

[182] Mayer, J., Roy, P., and Mitra, K.P. Relation between caloric intake, body weight, and physical work: studies in an industrial male population in West Bengal. *American Journal of Clinical Nutrition*, 4(2):169–175, 1956.

[183] Thomas, G., Bond, D.S., Hill, J.O., and Wing, R.R. The National Weight Control Registry: A study of "successful losers." *ACSM's Health & Fitness Journal*, 15(2):8–12, 2011.

[184] Catenacci, V.A., Odgen, L., Phelan, S., Thomas, J.G., Hill, J.O., Wing, R.R., and Wyatt, H.R. Dietary habits and weight maintenance success in high versus low exercisers in the National Weight Control Registry. *Journal of Physical Activity and Health*, 11(8):1540–1548, 2014.

[185] Ogden, L.G., Stroebele, N., Wyatt, H.R., Catenacci, V.A., Peters, J.C., Stuht, J., Wing, R.R., and Hill, J.O. Cluster analysis of the National Weight Control Registry to identify distinct subgroups maintaining successful weight loss. *Obesity*, 20(10):2039–2047, 2012.

Index

About the Author

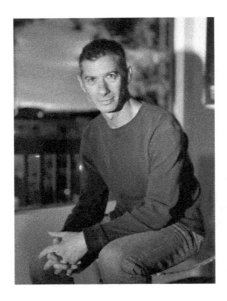

It started with a race around the track in sixth grade in Marlboro, New Jersey. Little did Jason know how much it would define his career and life. A Brooklyn, New York, native (you can take the boy out of Brooklyn, but you can't take Brooklyn out of the boy), he grew up playing baseball and soccer and running track. It was intoxicating. The passion that Jason found as a kid for the science of athletic performance (one of his earliest questions was how baseball pitchers throw curve balls) placed him on a yellow brick road that he still follows as a coach, exercise physiologist, author, speaker, and creator of the REVO2LUTION RUNNING™ certification program for coaches and fitness professionals around the world.

A TEDx speaker, Dr. Karp has given hundreds of international lectures and has been a featured speaker at most of the world's top fitness conferences and coaching clinics, including Asia Fitness Convention, Indonesia Fitness & Health Expo, FILEX Fitness Convention (Australia), US Track & Field and Cross Country Coaches Association Convention, American College of Sports Medicine Conference, IDEA World Fitness Convention, SCW Fitness MANIA, National Strength & Conditioning Association Conference, and CanFitPro, among others. He has been an instructor for USA Track & Field's level 3 coaching certification and for coaching camps at the US Olympic Training Center.

At age twenty-four, Dr. Karp became one of the youngest college head coaches in the country, leading the Georgian Court University women's cross-country team to the regional championship and winning honors as NAIA Northeast Region Coach of the Year. As a high school track and field and cross-country coach, he has produced state qualifiers and All-Americans. He is also the founder and coach of the elite developmental team, REVO2LUTION RUNNING ELITE.

A prolific writer, Jason is the author of nine other books: *The Inner Runner, Run Your Fat Off, Running a Marathon For Dummies, Sexercise, 14-Minute Metabolic Workouts, Running for Women, 101 Winning Racing Strategies for Runners, 101 Developmental Concepts & Workouts for Cross Country Runners,* and *How to Survive Your PhD.* He is also editor of the sixth edition of *Track & Field Omnibook.* He has more than four hundred articles published in numerous international coaching, running, and fitness trade and consumer magazines, including *Track Coach, Techniques for Track & Field and Cross Country, New Studies in Athletics, Runner's World, Running*

Times, Women's Running, Marathon & Beyond, IDEA Fitness Journal, Oxygen, PTontheNet.com, and *Shape,* among others. He also served as senior editor for Active Network.

Dr. Karp is a USA Track & Field nationally certified coach, has been sponsored by PowerBar and Brooks, and was a member of the silver-medal winning United States master's team at the 2013 World Maccabiah Games in Israel.

For his work and contributions to his industry, Jason was awarded the 2011 IDEA Personal Trainer of the Year (the fitness industry's highest award), is a two-time recipient of the President's Council on Sports, Fitness, & Nutrition Community Leadership Award (2014, 2019), and was a 2019 finalist for Personal Fitness Professional Trainer of the Year and 2020 finalist for Association of Fitness Studios Influencer of the Year.

Dr. Karp received his PhD in exercise physiology with a physiology minor from Indiana University in 2007, his master's degree in kinesiology from the University of Calgary in 1997, and his bachelor's degree in exercise and sport science with an English minor from Penn State University in 1995. He is currently pursuing his MBA at San Diego State University. His research has been published in the scientific journals *Medicine & Science in Sports & Exercise, International Journal of Sport Nutrition and Exercise Metabolism,* and *International Journal of Sports Physiology and Performance,* and he serves as a journal expert peer reviewer.

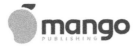

Mango Publishing, established in 2014, publishes an eclectic list of books by diverse authors—both new and established voices—on topics ranging from business, personal growth, women's empowerment, LGBTQ studies, health, and spirituality to history, popular culture, time management, decluttering, lifestyle, mental wellness, aging, and sustainable living.

We were recently named 2020's #1 fastest growing independent publisher by *Publishers Weekly*. Our success is driven by our main goal, which is to publish high quality books that will entertain readers as well as make a positive difference in their lives.

Our readers are our most important resource; we value your input, suggestions, and ideas. We'd love to hear from you—after all, we are publishing books for you!

Please stay in touch with us and follow us at:

Facebook: Mango Publishing
Twitter: @MangoPublishing
Instagram: @MangoPublishing
LinkedIn: Mango Publishing
Pinterest: Mango Publishing

Sign up for our newsletter at www.mango.bz and receive a free book!

Join us on Mango's journey to reinvent publishing, one book at a time.

CPSIA information can be obtained
at www.ICGtesting.com
Printed in the USA
LVHW091549220921
698251LV00006B/4

9 781642 503463